Crossfit

Introduce Crossfit Principles and Share Challenging Workout Routines

(Training Program for Body Strength and Conditioning through Extremely Challenging Workouts)

Norman Harty

I0089826

Published By **Cathy Nedrow**

Norman Harty

All Rights Reserved

Crossfit: Introduce Crossfit Principles and Share Challenging Workout Routines (Training Program for Body Strength and Conditioning through Extremely Challenging Workouts)

ISBN 978-1-7382986-2-4

No part of this guidebook shall be reproduced in any form without permission in writing from the publisher except in the case of brief quotations embodied in critical articles or reviews.

Legal & Disclaimer

The information contained in this book is not designed to replace or take the place of any form of medicine or professional medical advice. The information in this book has been provided for educational & entertainment purposes only.

The information contained in this book has been compiled from sources deemed reliable, and it is accurate to the best of the Author's knowledge; however, the Author cannot guarantee its accuracy and validity and cannot be held liable for any errors or omissions. Changes are periodically made to this book. You must consult your doctor or get professional medical advice before using any of the suggested remedies, techniques, or information in this book.

Table Of Contents

Chapter 1: Why Cross Fit For Seniors?

CrossFit, a form of practical health training, includes actions corresponding to sports activities in everyday lifestyles, at the side of squats, lunges, aerobic sports activities activities, and greater. It also consists of Olympic weightlifting, powerlifting, gymnastics, explosive movements, and specialized carrying sports like rope climbs and rowing. For those over the age of 60, CrossFit gives numerous potential fitness blessings.

One crucial problem of CrossFit is its strong feel of community, which fosters motivation and delight among individuals, as highlighted in a 2018 evaluate in Sports Medicine - Open. The lifestyle of resource within the CrossFit community is a massive detail in attracting and preserving individuals.

Longevity is a number one incentive for older adults considering CrossFit training. Numerous studies have verified that staying power training, immoderate-depth c language education (HIIT), and excessive-intensity beneficial training (HIFT) are associated with advanced longevity. A have a have a look at in the Journal of Aging Research observed that bodily active individuals can experience as an awful lot as seven more years of lifestyles.

For older adults who may be new to everyday workout, CrossFit's intensity might also moreover appear intimidating. However, scaling, a exercise that adjusts bodily sports to fit person competencies and comfort levels, lets in newcomers to take part properly.

According to a 2011 study in Deutsches Arzteblatt International, present day strength training in older adults is an effective way to combat muscle loss and hold motor characteristic, even at better intensities.

CrossFit's protection record is every other reassurance for older members. A 2018 evaluation inside the Orthopedic Journal of Sports Medicine endorsed that CrossFit education is notably strong compared to more conventional varieties of workout. Training maximum days of the week may additionally even lessen the threat of injury, ordinary with the same have a look at. Those who exercised much much less than 3 instances steady with week were at a higher risk of damage.

Furthermore, a 2020 have a examine inside the Journal of Human Kinetics concluded that the chance of damage in CrossFit is comparable to that during different sports activities activities. To lower the threat, new members are advocated to go through an model duration to beautify their technique, a key detail of CrossFit education.

Technique, often referred to as the "best of movement," is important to protection, performance, and effectiveness in CrossFit. Improving method is valuable to CrossFit technique, making sure that people can exercise correctly and successfully.

Scaling is the essential issue to introducing beginners to CrossFit. It includes adjusting exercising exercises or moves to in shape man or woman skills and desires, thinking about a gradual improvement. This is particularly essential even as learning new lifting patterns, as proper method is important, irrespective of age or health diploma.

Training in a set setting can beautify motivation and commitment through the years. A 2019 take a look at in PLoS One placed that the leisure and challenge of excessive-intensity useful education (HIFT) are strong motivators, and interpersonal relationships within the organisation end up more sizable as participation keeps. Another 2017 examine in BMJ Open Sport and Exercise Medicine strengthened the idea that group exercise lets in contributors meet endorsed physical hobby ranges.

The community issue of CrossFit makes it much more likely that people will preserve exercise and revel in it as they development. A 2017 have a study in BMC Geriatrics concluded that everyday employer exercise contributes to balanced fitness in older adults, enhancing their realistic health and everyday properly-being.

Concerns may moreover upward push up approximately institution fitness for people over 60, but workout plays a vital position in retaining fitness. A 2018 have a observe in Frontiers in Immunology decided that everyday workout complements immune feature and reduces the chance of each communicable and non-communicable illnesses, together with maximum cancers. Exercise has moreover been proven to mitigate the consequences of age-associated continual conditions.

As you could see, CrossFit offers numerous advantages for people aged 60 and above. It promotes sturdiness, bodily health, and a robust revel in of network, whilst also contributing to illness prevention. With right scaling, method improvement, and the help of the CrossFit network, older adults can efficiently and efficaciously engage on this shape of functional health schooling.

Debunking Myths and Misconceptions

CrossFit is a famous workout that some people misunderstand. People listen matters that could hold them from attempting CrossFit and getting its blessings. Here, we can treatment some commonplace wrong mind about CrossFit and give an reason behind the truth in an easy manner.

Myth 1: "I do no longer need to get too large."

Many people count on CrossFit will purpose them to appear to be bodybuilders. But the fact is, CrossFit may be adjusted to what you want. You do not have to get amazing huge. You can alternate your bodily video games to consciousness on staying lean and constructing staying power. CrossFit is set being purposeful and healthful, now not certainly consisting of masses of muscle.

Myth 2: "Cardio is greater essential than energy."

Some human beings anticipate CrossFit most effective cares approximately aerobic or electricity. But CrossFit does each in a high-quality way. It combines weightlifting, body weight sports, and cardio to make you ultra-modern fit. This permits you get ready for tremendous bodily sports sports.

Myth three: "I do no longer need to get damage."

People fear about getting damage doing CrossFit. Like any workout, there may be a few hazard. But if you do CrossFit proper, it's miles no longer more volatile than different sports. Doing the actions efficiently, adjusting the bodily video video games, and paying attention to your frame continues you secure. Trainers will manual you to do wearing sports in a safe way. CrossFit is ready making you more healthy, now not hurting you.

Myth four: "I'll reduce to rubble and be embarrassed."

Some people fear making mistakes and feeling embarrassed. Everyone starts somewhere, and no man or woman expects you to be best in advance than the whole lot. CrossFit is a supportive area. Trainers and others are there to assist and encourage you, not decide you. Making mistakes is a part of getting better, and those will admire your efforts.

Myth 5: "It's satisfactory for younger and suit human beings."

CrossFit is for every age and health levels. It's no longer only for more youthful or great healthful human beings. CrossFit can be adjusted for simply all people, regardless of in which you begin. It facilitates humans in their twenties, fifties, or perhaps older. Trainers will make sporting sports wholesome your abilties. Don't worry about your age or health degree; CrossFit is for everyone.

Myth 6: "It's too highly-priced."

Some say CrossFit charges too much. While it's far pricier than regular gyms, you get greater. CrossFit consists of schooling, planned workout routines, and a supportive community. Plus, better health is a protracted-term funding. Many human beings discover the assist and recommendation from CrossFit nicely properly well worth the price.

In brief, CrossFit has some misunderstandings, however the fact is simple: it's miles bendy, balanced, and welcomes every person. You can reap your health goals without annoying approximately getting harm or feeling embarrassed. People of each age and health ranges are welcome. By clearing up the ones myths, we're hoping greater people discover CrossFit and its blessings. Your CrossFit journey is precise, and fulfillment is possible.

Assessing Your Fitness Level

CrossFit is a exercise recurring that has grown in reputation in modern day years, attracting humans of numerous a while and fitness degrees. While CrossFit is often linked with rigorous physical video games and excessive-intensity schooling, it could moreover be a very powerful health utility for seniors.

However, growing a baseline evaluation is critical for older folks who want to begin or maintain CrossFit training. This baseline exam serves as an area to start in addition to a road map to steady and a hit schooling, ensuring that seniors may additionally enjoy the entire advantages of CrossFit on the equal time as fending off the chance of injury and overexertion.

Maintaining physical fitness and useful functionality as we age will become more essential for desired health and well-being. CrossFit is a splendid opportunity for seniors as it emphasizes useful bodily video games that reflect normal responsibilities, consequently improving energy, mobility, and cardiovascular fitness. A baseline assessment is vital for making the maximum of CrossFit schooling for numerous motives.

Safety First: One of the essential element reasons for doing a baseline evaluation is to make sure safety. CrossFit instructions are stated for his or her excessive intensity, which is probably horrifying for seniors who've not formerly participated in such strenuous physical interest. A baseline exam allows trainers to investigate a customer's contemporary health degree, understand any possible guidelines or fitness issues, and adapt this system to make certain it is secure and appropriate for the character. This proactive method aids within the prevention of injuries and overexertion, every of which might be greater common in older humans.

Goal Setting: A baseline evaluation offers an accurate photo of a person's present physical strengths and bounds. Both the instructor and the learner may create sensible and feasible fitness desires using this information. Seniors might also moreover have unique goals, which include developing balance, muscular energy, or cardiovascular health. The baseline evaluation is used to diploma progress and adapts the training software as required to meet those targets.

Individualized Training: CrossFit may be very customizable and may be tailored to each person's unique necessities and talents. A baseline evaluation permits trainers to alter workout workout routines to the man or woman's health degree with the beneficial resource of choosing appropriate sports activities and scaling the depth. For seniors, this could encompass changing an entire lot plenty much less strenuous joint sporting sports, integrating mobility schooling to enhance flexibility, and ensuring that physical video games are affordable however difficult.

Measuring Progress: Seeing development over the years is one of the maximum motivating additives of any health software. Seniors may additionally moreover diploma their improvement in energy, staying strength, flexibility, and stylish health with a baseline assessment. Regular reassessments may be executed to track development, making it much less tough to stay committed and encouraged. The feeling of success that comes from assembly and exceeding workout objectives may be particularly a laugh for seniors.

Preventing Plateaus: Without a baseline assessment, elders can also enjoy education plateaus Plateaus take place on the equal time as boom stops because of the truth the sporting events are not traumatic enough or because the identical sports are repeated without range. A baseline evaluation lets in running shoes to layout software program software that includes revolutionary overload, awesome motions, and pretty some modalities, keeping off plateaus and upsetting persistent improvement.

Increasing Confidence: Starting a fitness adventure, specially one as worrying as

CrossFit, is probably intimidating. Seniors, then again, might also additionally additionally gain self belief of their talents and trust the machine with a baseline evaluation. They are more likely to revel in a feel of success and pride in their accomplishments once they have a look at their adjustments and the way they've got evolved from their first assessment.

Health Monitoring: Health tracking is critical for older humans. The baseline examination may select out underlying fitness conditions or threat factors that would have an effect on education. Regular reviews may also moreover useful resource in the monitoring of changes in health, such as blood pressure, levels of cholesterol, or blood sugar degrees, deliberating early movement if required. CrossFit on foot footwear may also collaborate with healthcare professionals to make certain that seniors' fitness exercise routines are consistent with their medical necessities.

A baseline assessment is an crucial a part of CrossFit schooling for seniors. It permits for tailor-made training, assesses improvement, avoids plateaus, improves self assurance, and tests health. Seniors might also start on a CrossFit adventure that isn't always only difficult and fun, however furthermore acceptable to their specific requirements and capabilities with the useful resource of understanding and running inner their modern-day health diploma. A thorough baseline exam lays the muse for a a hit and happy CrossFit enjoy for elders, encouraging lengthy-time period health and nicely-being.

Chapter 2: Identifying Limitations and Goals

As you step into the area of CrossFit as a senior, it's far important to understand what you could do and what you want to reap. CrossFit has an entire lot of proper topics going for it, however it's far vital to recognize your limits and set clean dreams to make your schooling consistent and effective. Let's speak about why this subjects and the way you may navigate it to your CrossFit journey.

Knowing Your Limits

Let's first talk about how you can make a correct evaluation of your limits. This will help you put together well and make a plan that works flawlessly nicely for you.

Your Body: As we age, our our our bodies may not bypass as consequences. You should in all likelihood take a look at less flexibility, weaker muscle corporations, or a chunk a whole lot less endurance. It's ok! When planning your CrossFit workout exercises, reflect onconsideration on these items. Some bodily video games would in all likelihood want a tweak if they'll be too tough in your joints or muscular tissues.

Health Stuff: Seniors often have splendid fitness troubles. Things like arthritis, osteoporosis, or coronary coronary heart conditions want precise hobby even as planning your workouts. Make awesome to speak together together with your healthcare professionals to ensure CrossFit is right for you.

Past Injuries: Many people have had a bump or alongside the manner. If you've had injuries or surgical techniques, those need interest. Knowing your records lets in pick out wearing occasions that might not supply decrease lower back vintage pains.

Eating Right: Eating nicely is part of any health plan. Some human beings have specific diets due to fitness motives or personal options. Knowing what works for you lets in healthful up your vitamins collectively collectively with your CrossFit habitual.

In Your Head: Sometimes, it isn't pretty a lot the frame. Feeling irritating or unsure about sports is clearly ordinary. Recognizing the ones emotions we may want to going for walks shoes aid and cheer you on as you deal with demanding conditions.

Time Crunch: Life can get busy! If you've got were given circle of relatives stuff, artwork, or extraordinary subjects on your plate, your workout plan needs to in shape into it slow desk.

Setting Your Goals

You must want to set goals earlier than you start your CrossFit Exercise software. This will guide you on the form of physical video video games you do, the way you do them, and to what extent. These are some of the goals for which seniors collectively with you pick CrossFit wearing sports.

Better Daily Moves: Many seniors aim to stay lively and make regular responsibilities lots much less complicated. Things like going up stairs or wearing groceries grow to be smoother with improved balance, motion, and strength.

Heart Health Boost: A robust coronary heart is excessive to ordinary fitness. Setting desires like decrease blood strain or improved patience can hold your coronary coronary heart satisfied.

Muscle and Strength: Want to keep muscle corporations sturdy and prevent falls? Goals may likely encompass greater muscle organizations, toned muscle groups, or virtually feeling more potent in widespread.

Weight Watch: If retaining your weight in take a look at is a purpose, you're no longer by myself. Maintaining a healthy weight is vital for fashionable fitness and the way effects you could bypass spherical.

Ease the Pain: If you address chronic pain, your reason might be to locate comfort. CrossFit wearing sports activities can assist with the aid of boosting energy and versatility.

Mind Matters: CrossFit isn't always pretty much the body. It can do wonders for your thoughts too! Goals may additionally additionally embody much less stress, a better mood, or a sharper thoughts.

Connect with Others: Lots of seniors revel in the tremendous vibe of CrossFit. Goals can be making new pals, staying social, and feeling which includes you belong.

Hit Some Milestones: Feeling competitive? Setting private facts or possibly becoming a member of CrossFit competitions may be interesting desires to chase.

Putting It All Together

The magic in CrossFit for seniors takes location whilst your limits meet your goals. The utility works due to the fact it could modify physical activities to in shape what you need and want.

Matching Up: Knowing your limits allows you vicinity goals that make experience It continues subjects hard but viable, retaining you delivered on without overdoing it.

Adapting Workouts: Trainers can customise sporting events to paintings around your limits For example, in case your knees are a chunk finicky, they're capable of offer you with physical games that deliver a lift to without hurting

Seeing Progress: Recognizing limits manner you can degree development in a manner that makes feel for you It's all approximately moving in advance correctly.

Boosting Confidence: Acknowledging limits and hitting dreams, even small ones, can decorate yourself warranty. It makes achieving big desires down the street enjoy absolutely conceivable.

Staying Injury-Free: Customized wearing activities that do not forget your limits lower the hazard of getting damage This is greater important as we emerge as older and might be more vulnerable to accidents.

In the give up, information your limits and having easy goals make CrossFit first-rate for seniors. Understanding what your frame can take care of, managing fitness stuff well, and aiming for sensible but thrilling desires advocate you get all of the blessings of CrossFit without stressing out. It's all about locating that incredible balance so you can experience every step of your CrossFit journey!

Chapter 3: Preparing For Your Cross Fit Journey

Embarking on a CrossFit adventure as a senior is a transformative choice. Being organized, every mentally and bodily, is top. Understanding your goals, discussing fitness concerns with professionals, and deciding on the right fitness center with senior-pleasant programs guarantees a stable and first-class fitness adventure. Preparedness paves the path to achievement.

Choosing the Right CrossFit Gym or Space

Picking the proper CrossFit gymnasium subjects, mainly for seniors Where you figure out influences your protection, motivation, and conventional enjoy. When deciding on a health club for CrossFit, pay attention to 3 essential matters. These concerns must make a big distinction in how powerful and pleasant your exercise workouts are.

Accessibility and Location:

The location of the gym is important. It need to be near your home or interest. A community fitness center makes it much more likely you may persist with your exercise plan, it sincerely is essential for seniors. The gym need to additionally be clean to get into, with ramps, handrails, and no excessive steps. This ensures a secure and inviting region for all fitness tiers. For example, if you stay within the suburbs, look for a CrossFit health club internal a fifteen-minute stress. City dad and mom can also discover gyms close to public transit greater convenient.

Qualified Coaches:

The coaches at the gym play a massive issue to your CrossFit enjoy. Choose a fitness center with certified CrossFit teachers who have worked with older mother and father. These coaches want to understand the first-class wishes of seniors, like enhancing sporting activities and specializing in mobility and practical health. For example, look for taking walks footwear with credentials like CrossFit

Level 2 or specialized training for seniors. They want in an effort to percentage how they have got helped seniors attain their fitness desires.

Safety and Equipment:

Safety is crucial, specially for seniors. The gymnasium ought to have the right device for older human beings, like scaled sports activities, lighter weights, and mobility device. The facility must be clean, well-maintained, and observe protection rules to lessen the danger of injuries. For instance, pick out out gyms with unique machine for seniors, like resistance bands or lighter barbells. Check that the gym's gadget is regularly checked for safety.

Support and Community:

CrossFit is understood for its robust revel in of network. The perfect gym wants to encourage friendship, motivation, and range. Instructors and contributors should make seniors experience comfortable and supported. Pay interest to the health club's subculture. Does it have social activities, employer sports, or online beneficial resource businesses? Look for testimonials or success stories from seniors in their network.

Personalized Programs:

Everyone is specific, and seniors are not any exception. The gymnasium need to provide customized schooling plans that do not overlook your dreams, fitness diploma, and health issues. A one-period-fits-all method could now not paintings for seniors. Ask about the health club's approach to personalised programming. Do they look at your precise goals and goals? Can they percent examples of customized exercising plans for seniors?

Communication and Evaluation:

Good communication amongst coaches and customers is critical. Choose a fitness center in which coaches concentrate to your concerns, provide useful comments, and make crucial modifications. A gym that encourages open and ongoing communique ensures your training suits your desires and needs. Ask current humans approximately their research with coaches. Are teachers friendly, open to remarks, and inclined to regulate classes as desired?

Programming Balance:

A right CrossFit health club makes use of a balanced programming technique. To avoid plateaus and overuse problems, it need to include masses of actions, packages, and intensities. Seniors need a combination of aerobic interest, energy education, and mobility bodily sports for everyday health. Check the gymnasium's weekly or month-to-month programming calendar. It need to have hundreds of sports for a well-rounded fitness enjoy. Ask if they may be capable of offer examples of ordinary bodily sports for seniors.

Trial Period and Initial Evaluation:

Before becoming a member of, ask approximately an ordeal period or an preliminary evaluation. This helps you to enjoy the gymnasium's environment and training fashion. It additionally permits the gymnasium apprehend your health level and individual desires. For instance, many gyms offer each week or of unfastened trial instructions. Some offer a unfastened first assessment session to research your fitness and speak your dreams. Use the ones opportunities to attempt out the gym in advance than committing.

Adaptability and Scalability:

CrossFit is known for its scalability, it without a doubt is vital for seniors. Look for a gym that tailors physical sports on your modern fitness level. Coaches need to offer scaled options, allowing you to often boom depth as your power and ability develop. Ask coaches about their approach to scaling during a fitness center visit. They want to have the capacity to expose scaled workout routines designed for seniors with one-of-a-kind fitness abilities.

Health and Medical Considerations:

Seniors regularly have special health worries, and the health club must be privy to them. The health club desires to comprehend your scientific records, any gift situations, and any tablets you take. This guarantees the training software is steady and effective. Discuss your scientific records with the health club's personnel. They want to have the potential to expose how they have got custom designed exercise workouts for seniors with particular health troubles, like arthritis or diabetes.

Class Schedule and Availability:

Consider the elegance time table and availability on the health club. Seniors lead busy lives, so search for a health club with packages at instances that fit you. The gymnasium ought to be flexible, allowing you to change your schooling habitual as wanted. Check the gymnasium's elegance agenda and spot in the event that they provide morning, afternoon, or night intervals that healthful your schedule. Ask approximately their flexibility if you need to take away your bodily video games sometimes.

Pricing and Worth:

Finally, the membership rate need to in shape the offerings and assist supplied. While its miles tempting to pick out out out the most inexpensive gymnasium, it's miles equally essential to don't forget the fee you get. A gymnasium with expert education, personalised programming, and a pleasant environment can be properly worth your time and money. Compare the prices of gyms to your region and take a look at what everyone offers. Consider the splendid of education, customized help, and the gymnasium's music report with seniors.

Equipment and Attire for seniors

CrossFit, a shape of excessive-power health regular, can be an extremely good choice for seniors in search of to keep or beautify their physical fitness. But it is crucial to pick the right gear and clothes to make certain safety and effectiveness at some point of sporting events. This guide explores key troubles for tool and apparel in senior CrossFit training, presenting applicable examples and stressing the significance of creating knowledgeable alternatives.

Gear for Senior CrossFit Training:

1. Footwear: It's vital to position on flow into-training shoes that offer stability and assist for severa movements. Brands like Reebok and Nike provide alternatives appropriate for great foot shapes. Good shoes can help save you slips, useful resource your ankles, and enhance trendy stability.

2. Gloves and Wrist Wraps: Seniors handling joint ache or arthritis may additionally advantage from gloves and wrist wraps. These accessories offer more manual in your wrists and cushion your arms, lowering stress for the

duration of sports activities like push-united statesand kettlebell swings.

3. Weightlifting Belts: These belts provide essential decrease returned assist and help preserve proper form inside the direction of heavy lifting physical sports activities. Choose a properly-fitting, outstanding belt from legitimate manufacturers like Rogue Fitness or Harbinger.

4. Resistance Bands: Useful for reinforcing electricity and versatility, resistance bands are to be had in diverse stages suitable for seniors of diverse health stages. They may be used for physical games like pull-aparts, leg lifts, and stretching.

five. Foam Rollers and Mobility Aids: Maintaining flexibility and mobility is essential for seniors. Foam rollers, lacrosse balls, and mobility sticks can aid in style of movement and muscle tightness, making them effective for decent-up or cool-down workouts.

6. Specially Designed Barbells and Dumbbells: Some gyms provide barbells and dumbbells with smaller grips designed for seniors. These are much less complex to apply and offer a greater comfortable grip, lowering pressure at the hands and wrists.

Attire for Senior CrossFit Training:

1. Moisture-Wicking Clothing: Wear fitness center clothes fabricated from moisture-wicking fabric to maintain your body dry and comfortable throughout excessive sports. Brands like Under Armour and Lululemon offer some of suitable alternatives.

2. Compression Apparel: Compression shorts, leggings, or sleeves can useful aid in muscular assist, flow into, and recuperation, particularly for seniors with joint or muscular pain. Brands like 2XU and Zensah provide compression apparel for workout.

3. Breathable and Layered Clothes: Wear layered clothes that may be adjusted for comfort primarily based on the health club's

temperature. Moisture-wicking base layers and breathable tops can assist regulate temperature.

4. Proper Socks: Invest in moisture-wicking, padded CrossFit socks with arch guide to prevent blisters and pain for the duration of excessive bodily video games.

5. Supportive Sports Bras: Female seniors need to locate on supportive sports activities sports bras to lessen ache in the direction of sports activities regarding leaping or excessive-effect motions. Brands like Athleta and Panache offer sports sports sports bras with numerous ranges of manual.

6. Protective Gear: Depending on man or woman dreams, some seniors may additionally furthermore require extra protecting gear collectively with knee sleeves or elbow wraps to help joints at risk of ache or harm.

Chapter 4: Cross Fit Fundamentals

CrossFit embodies a holistic technique to fitness, emphasizing practical moves, scalability, consistent version, and intensity tailored to person wishes. It fosters a supportive community, encourages measurement and monitoring of development, and keeps a focal point on extended-term fitness and properly-being. These standards make CrossFit a bendy and effective health recurring for all.

CrossFit Principles and Philosophies

CrossFit isn't only a exercising ordinary; it's far a whole method that has changed the lives of many humans, no matter their age. Even even though CrossFit is thought for being immoderate, it's based totally mostly on thoughts that can be adjusted to satisfy the appropriate dreams and desires of seniors. By information and embracing the ones number one mind, older people can revel in the entire advantages of CrossFit at the same time as retaining themselves secure and nicely.

Everyday Movements

CrossFit is all approximately sensible actions—carrying activities that mimic normal sports activities. Squats, lifts, and jumps, as an instance, aren't high-quality useful however moreover amazing for building strength, flexibility, and stability. This is in particular essential for seniors as it at once contributes to their capability to perform every day duties independently and with greater ease. Functional actions, like reputation up from a chair without help or lifting a bag, assist seniors preserve their independence.

For example, incorporating squats into your CrossFit regular can significantly enhance your leg power, making it less tough to rise up from a sitting feature. These realistic movements can be tailor-made to your abilties and regularly superior to avoid overexertion.

Adjustability

Adjustability is a key aspect of CrossFit. This manner each workout can be custom designed on your health degree and private wishes. This is especially vital for seniors as it lets in them to begin at a comfortable diploma and improvement at their very personal pace. This ensures that CrossFit is available and regular for elders, reducing the danger of harm or overtraining.

To accommodate mobility boundaries, a scaled CrossFit exercising may also consist of step-united statesonto a decrease ground in place of container jumps. As your strength and self assurance expand, you could in the end improvement to the ordinary region soar movement.

Constant Variety

CrossFit prospers on the idea of regular range. These manner workout routines are severa to keep away from plateaus and promote popular health improvement. This range is useful for seniors because it annoying conditions the frame in new methods, enhancing cardiovascular health, electricity, and mobility without inflicting repetitive stress on joints and muscle businesses. The everyday exchange moreover continues the exercise interesting and attractive, essential for lengthy-time period commitment.

For seniors, this can contain alternating amongst electricity-based totally absolutely carrying occasions, aerobic-intensive instructions, and versatility-focused exercise routines. This numerous method helps older humans construct properly-rounded health and reduces the chance of pressure from repetitive movements.

Customized Intensity

While CrossFit is idea for its immoderate intensity, it is crucial to be aware that intensity is relative and may be adjusted to your fitness stage. To improve your health, you need to little by little growth your intensity. The venture for seniors is to discover a balance among pushing their limits for development and keeping off overexertion.

For instance, a senior can do a modified version of the famous CrossFit workout "Cindy," which includes frame weight actions like pull-ups, push-ups, and air squats. To hold safety even as gambling the benefits of the workout, the depth of this software can be adjusted thru reducing the extensive sort of repetitions and incorporating longer relaxation durations.

Supportive Community

CrossFit locations a strong emphasis on building a supportive community of like-minded people this experience of belonging fosters motivation, responsibility, and friendship. This manual community is important for seniors because it encourages everyday participation and a pleasing attitude towards exercising.

Group workout and a enjoy of belonging were shown in research to decorate adherence and motivation in older humans (BMJ Open Sport and Exercise Medicine, 2017). A CrossFit community not handiest gives workout companions however additionally partners with similar fitness desires.

Tracking Progress

CrossFit encourages measuring and monitoring progress. This concept is especially motivating for the aged. Older people can show tangible development over the years by manner of recording workout effects, monitoring weights lifted, or monitoring staying power degrees. The revel in of success and visible development may be in particular motivating for seniors, inspiring them to maintain their health adventure.

For instance, if a senior starts offevolved offevolved offevolved with a 10-pound dumbbell for a sure interest, tracking their improvement may moreover display that they could now without issues use a 15-pound dumbbell. These measurable adjustments not only beautify self assure however also act as smooth signs of bodily development.

Focus on Longevity

CrossFit takes a protracted-term approach to health. It's now not approximately immediately effects however approximately preserving lengthy-term health and happiness. Seniors are advised to view CrossFit as a fitness technique for the lengthy haul, reaping rewards them well into their golden years. CrossFit's emphasis on beneficial movements, energy, mobility, and cardiovascular health promotes durability and an fantastic high-quality of life.

The necessities and philosophies of CrossFit are adaptable and alternatively applicable for seniors. Following the requirements described, older people can embark on a fitness adventure that is solid, powerful, and exciting. It can display a valuable device in assisting seniors maintain their independence and average well-being as they age.

Functional Movements and Their Relevance

One of the reasons CrossFit has become famous as a exercise habitual is because of its reputation on useful movements. These sports sports are vital for seniors as they mimic actual-existence actions, helping to enhance electricity, mobility, and normal fitness. Understanding the ones moves is critical for growing powerful, consistent, and intention-oriented exercise packages for seniors within the context of CrossFit education.

The Importance of CrossFit Functional Movements for Seniors

The vital purpose of CrossFit for seniors is to beautify sensible fitness, letting them maintain independence and an energetic manner of life as they age. Functional movements are key to this intention as they goal muscle agencies and movement styles preferred for ordinary obligations. Squats (similar to getting up from a chair), pushing and pulling sports activities sports (like commencing doorways), and lunges (just like strolling and stair mountain climbing) are examples of such actions.

Injury Prevention: Seniors are extra vulnerable to accidents, in particular from falls and muscular imbalances. Functional moves, which includes complex sports activating multiple muscle corporations, help construct energy and coordination on the equal time as reducing the hazard of harm. For instance, the deadlift strengthens the decrease lower lower lower back and legs, enhancing stability and stability, vital for stopping falls.

Improved Range of Motion: Functional sports activities often require a entire kind of motion, important for joint fitness and versatility. Overhead lifts, squats, and kettlebell swings are examples of CrossFit carrying sports that take a look at and beautify joint mobility. This is mainly useful for the elderly, alleviating age-related stiffness and joint pain.

Adaptable Intensity: CrossFit schooling is notably scalable, allowing seniors to tailor wearing sports to their modern-day-day fitness diploma. Functional motions make a contribution to this scalability. For instance, a squat can be modified with the aid of adjusting intensity, adding assist, or the use of resistance bands, making it appropriate for seniors with numerous health degrees.

Core Strength and Stability: Core power is essential for correct posture, balance, and fundamental purposeful health. Exercises like planks, farmer's supply, and remedy ball slams aim middle muscles, improving balance and decreasing the threat of another time damage. A sturdy center is essential for seniors to maintain an upright posture and assist their spine.

Cardiovascular Health: CrossFit for seniors frequently includes functional exercising exercises that boom coronary coronary coronary heart charge and enhance cardiovascular fitness. Activities like rowing, cycling, and burpees art work the cardiovascular tool, improving staying power and stamina. This is important for seniors to preserve power and coronary coronary heart health.

Examples of Functional Movements in CrossFit for Seniors

Air Squat: These important practical movement mimics sitting and developing from a chair, helping seniors preserve leg energy, balance, and the capability to take a seat and stand independently.

Kettlebell Swings: A dynamic exercising that engages the hips, decrease again, and legs, kettlebell swings raise coronary coronary coronary heart rate and improve energy and explosiveness, beneficial for lifting and carrying gadgets.

Push-ups: Functional for strengthening the chest, shoulders, and triceps, push-united stateshold higher body strength, vital for obligations like lifting and wearing out immoderate.

Farmer's Carry: Walking with weights in each hand enhances grip, middle stability, and popular balance, simulating sports activities along with sporting groceries.

Box Jumps: Improving decrease frame explosiveness and coordination, adjustable container jumps are suitable for seniors aiming to beautify leg strength and strength.

Medicine Ball Throws: Forceful motions the use of the complete frame assist keep or growth seniors' functionality to elevate, carry, and circulate devices.

Chapter 5: Beginner and Advanced Cross Fit Exercises

CrossFit exercising exercises may be adjusted that will help you preserve your strength, flexibility, and ordinary fitness. Here are a few CrossFit bodily sports for seniors, together with particular commands at the manner to do them accurately and successfully:

Sample Beginner CrossFit Exercises

1. Air Squats:

Stand along with your ft shoulder-width aside.

Keep your chest up, shoulders again, and middle engaged.

Lower your body by means of manner of using bending your hips and knees.

Keep a instantly line amongst your knees and toes.

Lower yourself until your thighs are parallel to the floor.

Return to the starting feature by the use of pressing thru your heels.

Note: You can use a chair or a wall for help if needed. Focus on shape and manipulate in place of depth.

2. Kettlebell Swings:

Stand along side your feet shoulder-width apart and feet have become out slightly.

Hold a kettlebell inside the the the front of you with each arms, hands outstretched.

Hinge at your hips, pushing your buttocks decrease decrease returned while maintaining your spine unbiased.

Swing the kettlebell among your thighs, and then press your hips in advance to swing it as a brilliant deal as shoulder pinnacle.

Control the drop and swing once more.

Note: Start with a moderate kettlebell to make sure proper form. This exercise objectives the hips and middle.

3. Box Step-Ups:

Stand at the facet of your feet hip-width aside in the the front of a robust field or step Step onto the world via setting one foot on it and pushing through the heel Stand tall at the field, making sure your knee does no longer increase past your toes.

Return to your beginning position via taking a step back.

Note: You can modify the field pinnacle for your consolation diploma and growth the hassle regularly.

4. Wall Push-Ups:

Stand going through a wall, approximately arm's length away.

Place your fingers at shoulder top at the wall, flat.

Step your ft lower lower returned, maintaining a proper away line together along with your frame.

Lower your chest within the route of the wall by means of the usage of the usage of bending your elbows.

Return to the start function.

Note: Wall push-usaare a mild manner to construct pinnacle frame electricity, and you could modify the distance to differ the intensity.

5. Planks:

Start at the ground, elbows really under your shoulders.

Extend your legs at the back of you whilst retaining your body without delay.

Engage your center and hold your posture.

Breathe evenly and motive to keep the plank feature for 15-30 seconds to start with, often growing through the years.

Note: You can do a changed plank on your knees for a whole lot less effort. Focus on maintaining a without delay posture.

6. Seated Leg Raises:

Sit on a strong chair, decrease lower back upright, and feet flat at the ground.

Hold the chair's facets for balance.

Lift one leg directly out in the front of you, parallel to the floor.

Hold for some seconds earlier than decreasing it all over again.

Repeat with the alternative leg.

This workout improves leg electricity and stability, making it an awesome preference for seniors.

7. Dumbbell Rows:

Sit on a sturdy bench or chair and keep a dumbbell in a unmarried hand.

Put your opposite knee and hand at the bench for useful useful resource.

Maintain a right away once more and allow the dumbbell hold close down.

Squeeze your shoulder blades together as you pull the load towards your hip.

Return the dumbbell to its starting function and repeat.

This exercise improves pinnacle-frame power and may be completed with lighter weights.

8. Banded Pull-Aparts:

Stand together with your toes shoulder-width aside.

Hold a resistance band with each hands inside the the the front of you, arms outstretched.

Pull the band apart by using using extending your arms out to the rims and pushing your shoulder blades collectively.

Return on your start line.

Note: Banded pull-apart are an superb exercising for growing shoulder mobility and energy.

Always are searching for advice from a healthcare professional or fitness professional earlier than starting any exercise application, particularly if you have pre-present day clinical problems. Begin with mild weights or resistance bands and regularly growth the intensity as you gain self notion for your actions. CrossFit carrying occasions for seniors require safety, right method, and revolutionary improvement.

Advanced CrossFit Exercises for seniors

1. Dumbbell Goblet Squats:

Stand collectively together with your feet apart, as good sized as your shoulders.

Hold a dumbbell near your chest with every hand.

Keep your chest up and tighten your belly muscle mass.

Bend your hips and knees to decrease your body whilst retaining the dumbbell close to your chest.

Go as little as you without problems can even as preserving correct shape.

Stand lower back up through pushing thru your heels.

Note: This exercise provides weight in your squats, making your leg muscle groups paintings tougher. Start with mild dumbbells and step by step use heavier ones.

2. Medicine Ball Slams:

Stand along with your ft hip-width apart, protective a remedy ball with each hand above you.

Engage your belly muscular tissues and enlarge your fingers to slam the ball forcefully into the floor.

Bend your knees a bit as you seize the ball at the soar to take in the effect.

Repeat the slamming motion.

Note: Medicine ball slams art work your whole body, focusing on center and better body energy. Begin with a slight medication ball and interest on right approach. ·

3. Ring Rows:

Set up gymnastic earrings at chest degree.

Hold one ring in each hand with arms coping with each particular.

Walk your toes ahead and lean lower again to create tension at the jewelry.

Keep your frame right now and pull your chest in the route of the jewelry.

Return to the beginning characteristic and repeat.

Note: Ring rows target the higher body, mainly the over again and biceps. Adjust the angle by way of using shifting your toes for added or tons much less trouble.

4. The Farmer's Walk:

Hold a dumbbell or kettlebell in each hand with the aid of manner of way of your aspects.

Stand tall at the side of your chest up and shoulders lower lower back.

Walk purposefully, taking controlled steps at the same time as keeping proper posture.

Continue for a set quantity of time or distance.

Note: The Farmer's Walk builds grip strength and works more than one muscle companies. Start with slight weights and regularly increase as you get more potent.

five. Burpees:

Begin along side your toes hip-width apart.

Place your fingers at the floor and reduce yourself right into a squat role.

Move right right into a plank feature together together with your ft.

Do a push-up or hold the plank function.

Return your toes to the squat feature.

Extend your fingers upward and bounce into the air.

Note: Burpees are a entire-frame workout that enhances cardiovascular health and energy. Start with a changed model, like skipping the frenzy-up, and development to the overall burpee.

6. Toes-to-Bar:

Hang from a pull-up bar together with your palms truely prolonged.

Bring your toes up towards the bar whilst attractive your middle.

Aim to touch your feet to the bar.

Lower your legs lower back to the start characteristic with manage.

Repeat the motion.

Note: Toes-to-bar mission your middle strength and grip. Begin with knee raises or leg lifts and improve to toes-to-bar.

7. Double-Unders (Jump Rope):

Hold a leap rope in each hand.

For every leap, spring off the floor and swing the rope beneath your toes twice.

Keep your arms snug and bounce with a mild, steady soar.

Increase the fee of the rope for extra tough repetitions.

Double-unders beautify cardiovascular health and coordination. Start with single jumps and development to double-unders while you are prepared.

Always prioritize protection and proper form. Consult a fitness expert to determine if those superior physical activities are appropriate in your cutting-edge health level. As you advantage self warranty and power, regularly increase the depth and weight. Warm up and funky down earlier than and after each exercising, and pay interest to your frame, adjusting routines as had to save you damage.

Chapter 6: Scaling and Modifying Workouts

Adapting sports activities for seniors is important to make certain stable and effective exercising. Scaling and enhancing exercises cater to individual capabilities and desires. Lighter weights, reduced repetitions, and much less hard actions save you overexertion and restrict the danger of harm

these modifications well known the sort of older adults' health stages and assist them hold their health and independence. By making bodily games handy and a laugh, seniors can hopefully encompass physical activity, reaping the severa advantages it offers as they age.

Adapting CrossFit WODs (Workout of the Day) for Seniors

CrossFit is concept for its excessive exercising workouts and cognizance on useful movements. Even even though it is regularly associated with more youthful, greater athletic individuals, it is able to additionally be beneficial for seniors. However, one period does not in shape all, so it's far important to alter Cross Fit carrying sports to make sure your safety and decorate your overall performance.

Why Adapt Cross Fit for seniors?

CrossFit is ready scaling, because of these customizing wearing activities on your modern-day health degree and capability. For seniors, it's miles even greater important to tailor CrossFit bodily sports to their specific needs. Seniors frequently face demanding conditions like reduced muscular tissues, decrease bone density, decreased joint flexibility, and numerous health issues. So, carrying occasions need to be adjusted to cope with those elements whilst nevertheless imparting an effective training plan.

Here are some key factors to consider and mind for boosting CrossFit exercising workouts for seniors:

Individual Evaluation: Before growing a custom designed CrossFit software, a private assessment is vital. This consists of reviewing your scientific statistics, any bodily regulations or accidents, and your current-day fitness diploma. This information is critical for developing a custom designed method that addresses your unique desires and desires.

Low-Impact Movements: Because seniors' joints and bones are greater touchy, excessive-effect moves may not be suitable. Focus on low-impact exercising workouts like step-ups, seated leg lifts, and resistance band education. These sports offer blessings with minimum hazard of damage.

Functional Movements: CrossFit emphasizes practical actions that mimic ordinary obligations. These actions can be especially useful for seniors, improving energy and mobility for each day sports. Examples encompass air squats, kettlebell swings, and push-ups.

Reduced Weight Intensity: Heavy weights can boom the risk of harm in seniors. Start with lighter weights and little by little boom resistance as energy improves. For instance, use a mild-weight treatment ball or frame weight squats in place of a heavy barbell lower back squat.

Scaled Intensity: Reduce exercising depth for seniors. Modify training time and embody longer rest periods. For example, a excessive-intensity workout with short relaxation periods can be adjusted to have longer relaxation intervals for recovery.

Stressing Mobility: Senior fitness want to attention on mobility. Many seniors have limited fashion of movement and versatility. Modify CrossFit sports to encompass mobility physical games like dynamic stretching or yoga.

Functional Training Equipment: Use useful education device like resistance bands, stability balls, and suspension running shoes to conform CrossFit for seniors. These tools help seniors carry out physical sports because it need to be and efficaciously.

Monitoring Heart Rate: Seniors have to be privy to their coronary heart fee for the duration of exercise. Using heart fee video show devices guarantees they function at a strong intensity degree for his or her age institution.

Regular Assessments: Regularly assessment development to ensure custom designed CrossFit physical games align with fitness dreams. This lets in for software adjustments to save you plateaus.

Educated Coaches: CrossFit coaches dealing with seniors ought to gain knowledge of in senior health. They want attention of the unique desires and annoying situations seniors face to format and supervise customized exercise exercises.

Adapting CrossFit physical video games for seniors is ready ensuring they're succesful to take part efficiently and experience the advantages it offers. Seniors can also interact in CrossFit in a manner that promotes health, power, and commonplace nicely-being through specializing in individual tests, low-impact actions, purposeful sports activities, reduced weight intensity, scaled intensity, mobility, useful schooling tool, coronary heart charge tracking, everyday tests, and knowledgeable coaches.

Here's an instance of an tailor-made CrossFit exercise for seniors:

WOD: Senior Strength and Mobility

Warm-up: 5 mins of low-intensity workout (collectively with desk sure cycling).

Mobility sports: dynamic stretches focusing on key joints like hips, shoulders, and ankles.

Primary Workout:

Air squats: 3 sets of ten to 12 repetitions the usage of a balance ball for stability.

Seated leg lifts: three gadgets of 10-12 repetitions using ankle weights.

Resistance band rows: 3 units of 10-12 repetitions.

Rest: 60 seconds amongst units.

Cool-down: Gentle stretching and thorough respiratory carrying sports.

Monitoring coronary heart charge to make certain it remains inside a regular range.

This tailored workout consists of low-impact actions, mobility artwork, and resistance physical sports activities even as reducing depth to fulfill seniors' goals. It enhances electricity and mobility, allowing seniors to guide an active and healthful manner of lifestyles.

Safety and Injury Prevention

CrossFit education is thought for its hard physical video video games, making it a exquisite fitness desire for reinforcing favored fitness and fitness. Seniors are also spotting the blessings of CrossFit's awareness on realistic activities. However, like several exercising, older people need to prioritize safety and injury prevention. In this guide, we're capable of find out key protection issues, damage prevention strategies, and applicable examples to help seniors enjoy the advantages of CrossFit with out setting themselves at danger.

Consultation with Healthcare Professionals: Before beginning CrossFit, talk over together along with your healthcare practitioner, mainly when you have pre-modern scientific problems or injuries. Your clinical doctor's advice can help discover capability dangers and create a custom designed fitness plan considering your unique health problems. For instance, when you have a facts of decrease decrease lower back issues, speak over with an orthopedic professional to speak about appropriate bodily video games and adjustments.

Proficient Trainers: Choose a in a characteristic and skilled CrossFit instructor who is familiar with senior-precise fitness components. They ought with a view to create age-suitable exercise exercises, offer guidance on relevant approach, and be aware about age-related health issues. An skilled CrossFit teacher might in all likelihood endorse beginning with lighter weights and specializing in enhancing approach before growing depth.

Warm-Up and Cool-Down Routines: Prioritize remarkable sufficient warmness-up and cool-down sporting activities for harm prevention, particularly as an older character. Warming up prepares your frame for hobby, at the equal time as cooling down reduces the chance of muscular pain and harm. For seniors, a warm-up can also encompass slight cardiovascular sports activities and dynamic stretching, observed by way of static stretching and foam rolling for cooling down.

Proper Scaling: Exercises want to be scaled to your fitness diploma to keep away from pushing beyond your capability. Trainers can alter bodily video games to strengthen inclined regions grade by grade. For instance, if fashionable push-united states of america of the us of americaare difficult, running shoes can also start with incline or wall push-americaand improvement to normal push-america strength improves.

Progressive Overload: A properly-constructed CrossFit software must include progressive overload, grade by grade developing the depth of sports to prevent overuse accidents. Seniors can also moreover begin with lighter weights and shorter training durations, grade by grade developing the load and period as they come to be extra comfortable and more potent.

Listening in your Body: Pay interest in your frame at the same time as you workout. Don't forget about ache or soreness. Stop the interest if some thing does not feel right and are looking for for advice from a trainer to avoid greater excessive accidents. For example, if you studies knee ache for the duration of squats, it's crucial to address the trouble in preference to ignoring the pain.

Nutrition and Hydration: Maintain a properly-balanced weight loss program and stay hydrated to guide bodily hobby and prevent accidents. Dehydration can reason muscular cramps, growing the chance of damage. Seniors ought to prioritize hydration in advance than, at some point of, and after CrossFit exercises.

Rest and Recovery: Incorporate rest and recovery days into your health ordinary. Seniors may additionally need more time between superb sports activities sports to allow their our our bodies to get better. If experiencing muscular pain, seniors ought to take enough time to heal, doubtlessly lowering workout frequency and intensity till organized to resume complete training.

Constant Communication: Maintain open conversation together together with your trainers. Feel snug addressing any issues or pain, permitting jogging footwear to make essential modifications in your schooling. For instance, if a senior research hip pain at some point of squats, speaking this to the teacher lets in changes to be made, together with enhancing squat approach or deciding on opportunity physical sports activities.

CrossFit schooling can be effective for seniors, but it must be approached with warning and a focal point on damage prevention. By following the instructions right right here, seniors can experience the advantages of CrossFit at the identical time as minimizing the danger of damage. With the ones worries in vicinity, seniors can embark on a CrossFit adventure that enables their health, nicely-being, and strength.

Training Programs for Seniors

CrossFit is for all of us, which encompass seniors. Though it is appeared for more more youthful human beings, it may be useful for older folks too. However, for seniors to engage correctly and efficaciously in CrossFit, particular schooling plans are crucial. This manual focuses on the crucial factors of CrossFit training for seniors, emphasizing safety, adaptability, and accomplishing desires. We'll use examples and references to help you recognize higher.

Understanding Your Needs and Limits

Before beginning any CrossFit software, it's miles critical to evaluate your unique wishes, competencies, and obstacles. This consists of a systematic checkup, a take a look at of your mobility and versatility, and an assessment of your cutting-edge-day-day fitness diploma. This evaluation paperwork the premise for developing a personalized education software program application.

Imagine you're a sixty five-12 months-vintage guy trying to attempt CrossFit. The evaluation well-known restrained mobility to your hips and shoulders because of past accidents, however your cardiovascular situation is adequate. This records permits the trainer layout a utility focusing on mobility carrying sports and scaled movements that may not worsen your past problems.

Setting Goals and Monitoring Progress

Seniors, like everyone else, need to set precise and viable exercising desires, which includes improving typical electricity, balance, agility, or flexibility. Setting goals now not pleasant offers motivation but moreover helps layout a education software program aligned with those desires. Seniors can artwork with their coaches to growth short-term and extended-time period goals, giving their CrossFit adventure cause.

For example, a 70-12 months-antique's aim might be to beautify stability and decrease the risk of falling. Exercises specializing in stability and coordination, like unmarried-leg squats or balancing board drills, can be protected. They can diploma improvement with the resource of gauging their capability to perform those sports activities extra efficiently over the years.

Adapting Workouts and Scaling Exercises

Adapting exercising exercises for your fitness diploma and bodily obstacles is essential. CrossFit walking shoes have to be expert in enhancing sports so seniors can take part appropriately at the same time as nevertheless experiencing this tool's intensity.

For example, a 60-12 months-antique suffering with traditional pull-u.S.May use resistance bands or ring rows alternatively. These scaled bodily sports activities assist paintings toward the goal of doing unassisted pull-u.S.A.Without pressure or damage.

Progressive Overload and Variety

Seniors' training plans ought to encompass progressive overload, gradually developing workout depth to promote ongoing power and staying power profits. Variety ensures their fitness degrees stay severa and that they get a properly-rounded exercising software.

A sixty eight-12 months-antique beginning with slight-weight kettlebell swings would probable frequently increase the burden as they benefit skillability. Introducing new sports like squats, deadlifts, or vicinity jumps provides variety and engages super muscle groups.

Monitoring Health and Recovery

Regular fitness test-ins, alongside side blood strain and coronary heart fee, assist strolling footwear and contributors stay on pinnacle of any changes which could require software versions. Seniors also can moreover need extra time for relaxation and recovery than more youthful human beings.

For example, a 72-one year-vintage with a facts of hypertension want to have regular blood strain tests. If any troubles upward push up, the schooling software may be adjusted to encompass more low-intensity bodily sports and stress-good deal approaches.

Social and Community Involvement

CrossFit for seniors is not pretty tons bodily blessings; the social and network additives are crucial too. Participating in a collection placing can be motivating, fostering camaraderie and duty. The CrossFit network offers emotional guide, improving the general enjoy.

Consider a 67-12 months-antique becoming a member of a CrossFit magnificence; they discover motivation and companionship among friends, sharing evaluations and fostering a outstanding environment. This experience of belonging motivates them to live steady in schooling.

Regular Reassessments

Periodic reassessments are crucial to alter this device as wanted and set up new dreams. Fitness tiers, health situations, and targets can also moreover trade over the years, and reassessments ensure the schooling remains relevant on your evolving wishes.

For example, a 75-year-vintage may also additionally find out advanced energy at some point of a reassessment, prompting a trade in the schooling software software to attention greater on retaining and growing their newfound power.

CrossFit may be a terrific fitness software program software for seniors while tailor-made to their particular desires. Prioritizing protection, aim planning, scalability, progressive overload, range, fitness tracking, community involvement, and periodic evaluation in custom designed training applications offers an inclusive and a success exercising revel in. This approach improves physical and intellectual properly-being in later life, making sure a satisfied and sustainable fitness adventure for seniors.

Chapter 7: Building Strength and Endurance

In CrossFit training for seniors, the point of interest is on constructing power and stamina. The cause is to enhance sensible fitness and ordinary health as opposed to placing private records. Strength physical video video games are useful for keeping muscle groups and bone density, critical for growing older our our bodies. Endurance physical sports contribute to higher cardiovascular fitness and stamina, vital for an active lifestyles. By prioritizing the ones additives, seniors can revel in improved mobility, reduced danger of harm, and a higher exceptional of existence. The adaptable technique of CrossFit guarantees that seniors can assemble strength and staying power correctly and correctly.

Strength Training for Seniors

Maintaining physical fitness becomes more critical as we age so one can preserve a first rate best of life and independence. Strength training is an important thing of an everyday fitness software program software for older human beings. It improves not sincerely muscular increase and power, but additionally bone density, balance, and fashionable useful ability. Here, we're capable of check the significance of energy education for older human beings, which incorporates its a couple of advantages, essential problems, and pertinent instances or references.

The Importance of Strength Training for Senior Citizens

Aging is associated with a number of physiological modifications, which encompass a natural drop in muscle companies, known as sarcopenia, and a decrease in bone density. These changes also can furthermore result in some of age-related health troubles, such as frailty, an extended chance of falling, and osteoporosis. Strength schooling, furthermore called resistance training, can be an effective method for preventing the outcomes of having older.

Muscular Mass and Strength: One of the maximum glaring benefits of electricity education for older males and females is the maintenance and increase of muscular mass and electricity. This now not quality enhances movement but additionally makes it much much less tough to do each day obligations. When muscular power is maintained, for instance, carrying groceries or mountain climbing stairs turns into more capability.

Bone Health: Strength training locations the bones under stress, which evokes the formation of recent bone tissue and will boom bone density. This is specifically crucial for older men and women because it lowers the hazard of osteoporosis and fractures. Weight-bearing sports, which encompass squats and deadlifts, are terrific examples of bone-healthful electricity education sports activities.

Many energy education sports require balance and balance, which may be crucial for lowering falls in older people. Single-leg sports, which includes step-americaor lateral leg lifts, name for balance and coordination, which allows to decrease the chance of falling.

Metabolism and Weight Control: Strength schooling will growth muscular mass, which may moreover moreover improve metabolism. Older parents with a more metabolic price can also furthermore higher manipulate their weight and lower their danger of obesity-associated health problems.

The potential to preserve electricity and mobility through electricity training has an instantaneous impact on an older person's independence. Physical power is at once associated with the self notion to conduct normal responsibilities independently, inclusive of getting internal and out of a chair or bathtub.

Mental Health: Strength education gives cognitive advantages. It can also moreover raise temper and alleviate anxiety and depression symptoms. Endorphins, which may be herbal temper elevators, are released after exercise, particularly strength schooling.

Key Considerations for Strength Training in Older Adults

While there are numerous advantages to energy training for older parents, there are some essential factors to maintain in mind to guarantee protection and achievement.

Visit a Healthcare Professional: Before beginning any fitness application, older people, especially human beings with underlying health issues, ought to visit a healthcare practitioner or scientific physician. They can also advocate on unique workout exercises which may be each safe and suitable.

Proper Form and Technique: Proper shape and approach are crucial for retaining off harm. To boom correct exercising technique and assure protection, it's miles top notch to have interaction with a expert fitness trainer, specifically one that has expertise with older parents.

Begin slowly: Older folks want first of all a modest degree of resistance and frequently growth it as they develop. Excessive strive or the use of huge weights too rapid would possibly bring about muscular strains or different issues.

Exercise Variety: A properly-rounded power education utility want to embody physical games that concentrate on numerous muscle groups. This allows to avoid overuse injuries and ensures that muscle mass increase in a balanced manner.

Recovery Time: Adequate relaxation and restoration time amongst power education periods is vital. When in comparison to more more youthful humans, older folks may also moreover take extra time to get nicely.

Nutrition and Hydration: Adequate nutrients and hydration are critical for muscle development and recuperation. Adequate protein intake is specially crucial for aged folks who want to maintain their muscular mass.

Tracking Progress: Keep a log of your development, along with the weights lifted, repetitions, and devices. Tracking development no longer most effective maintains motivation immoderate however additionally offers a clean photograph of improvement.

Cardiovascular Conditioning and Metabolic Conditioning

Cardiovascular Conditioning and Metabolic Conditioning: Tailoring CrossFit Training for Optimal Senior Fitness

CrossFit is renowned for its dynamic and all-encompassing approach to health, pushing human beings to their limits for ordinary fitness development. While often associated with excessive-intensity carrying events and weightlifting, CrossFit incorporates a essential detail that holds big importance for humans of all ages, particularly seniors: cardiovascular and metabolic health.

Cardiovascular conditioning, generally referred to as aerobic or cardio workout, is a essential thing of any whole fitness software application. It specializes in improving the frame's capability to transport oxygen to running muscle companies and successfully get rid of waste products. Metabolic conditioning, but, includes excessive-intensity, entire-body exercising routines designed to elevate the frame's metabolic rate, leading to extra green calorie burning and average fitness improvement. The amalgamation of those functions inner CrossFit training can show tremendously beneficial, especially for seniors.

Cardiovascular Conditioning for Seniors in CrossFit

Cardio sports activities collectively with strolling, cycling, rowing, and jumping rope are vital for seniors to maintain heart health, lung feature, and normal staying power. Here are key worries regarding cardiovascular conditioning in CrossFit for seniors:

Heart Health: Engaging in everyday cardiovascular exercising reduces the risk of coronary coronary heart illness, lowers blood pressure, and contributes to regular cardiovascular nicely-being. This is particularly essential for seniors, who may be greater susceptible to cardiac issues.

Lung Function: Cardio wearing sports activities enhance lung functionality, facilitating superior oxygen exchange and decreasing breathlessness, a common issue for growing older people.

Endurance: Cardiovascular workout enhances staying power, making every day sports more possible for seniors and improving normal performance in other CrossFit carrying sports.

Mood and Mental Health: Beyond bodily blessings, aerobic exercise has been associated with advanced mood and intellectual fitness, addressing crucial factors of normal nicely-being in seniors.

Adaptability: CrossFit's flexibility permits seniors to select low-impact aerobic sports activities, which includes desk sure biking or brisk strolling, tailor-made to their health levels and bodily constraints.

Metabolic Conditioning for Seniors in CrossFit

Metabolic conditioning, often referred to as MetCon, involves excessive-intensity, whole-body bodily games that project the frame's metabolic methods. Activities like kettlebell swings, area jumps, burpees, and rowing are commonly integrated. Here's why MetCon is particularly beneficial for seniors engaged in CrossFit:

Efficient Calorie Burning: MetCon notably increases the body's calorie burn fee, assisting seniors in weight control—a vital consideration given the capability health affects of greater weight in later years.

Muscle Building: MetCon sporting activities engage multiple muscle groups, promoting muscular improvement and prolonged electricity. Preserving muscle organizations is crucial for seniors to prevent age-related muscle loss (sarcopenia).

Metabolism Boost: High-depth durations in MetCon physical sports activities elevate the body's metabolic charge, important to persevered calorie burning even after the exercising concludes—a tremendously powerful approach for simple health enhancement.

Functional Strength: MetCon exercises are designed to imitate normal sports, contributing to advanced useful energy and agility, crucial for seniors aiming to preserve independence and carry out daily obligations with out issues.

Time Efficiency: MetCon exercising workouts, normally short but excessive, offer an tremendous opportunity for seniors with busy schedules, permitting them to acquire an entire-frame exercising in only a few mins.

The Synergy of Cardiovascular and Metabolic Conditioning

The mixture of cardiovascular and metabolic health is critical to CrossFit schooling for seniors. Cardio physical games prepare the body for the depth of MetCon, whilst MetCon provides variety and delight to habitual cardio exercise sporting events. The synergy among those components yields severa ordinary benefits:

Improved Overall Fitness: The synergy amongst cardio and MetCon contributes to a holistic improvement in everyday fitness. Seniors can count on upgrades in cardiovascular health, muscular electricity, staying electricity, and metabolism.

Weight Management: The more calorie burn from MetCon, coupled with the coronary heart-wholesome effects of aerobic exercise, aids seniors in efficiently dealing with their weight—an essential trouble in addressing age-associated health troubles.

Reduced Risk of Chronic Disease: CrossFit sporting sports that incorporate each cardiovascular and metabolic conditioning have the functionality to lower the threat of persistent ailments at the side of diabetes, high blood strain, and metabolic syndrome.

Better Quality of Life: As seniors witness improvements in health, muscular electricity, and cardiovascular health, their stylish outstanding of lifestyles is probably to decorate. This translates into the potential to pursue interests, travel, and spend time with cherished ones without feeling constrained with the useful resource of physical barriers.

Community and Support: The CrossFit network plays a crucial position in motivating seniors to stay regular with their schooling. Being part of a supportive organization can assist them stay dedicated to regular bodily sports activities, fostering a experience of belonging and encouragement.

Cardiovascular and metabolic conditioning shape critical additives of CrossFit education for seniors. These factors contribute to stepped forward coronary heart fitness, lung function, patience, muscular electricity, and regular fitness. The versatility of CrossFit permits seniors to comply their bodily video games to their specific desires and constraints, making it a tremendous health application. The blessings of incorporating those conditioning additives are manifold, providing seniors with the competencies had to keep a excessive degree of physical and intellectual nicely-being as they age. The holistic technique of CrossFit guarantees that seniors can revel in an active and pleasant way of existence in their later years.

Chapter 8: Nutrition and Recovery

Eating proper and looking after your self are key factors of a a fulfillment CrossFit adventure for seniors such as you. A properly healthy dietweight-reduction plan with plenty of lean proteins, entire grains, and fruits and greens gives your body the energy it wishes for exercise exercises and lets in your muscle companies heal.

It's crucial to drink enough water, and meals with protein and anti-inflammatory houses can useful resource your healing. Getting sufficient rest and sleep is important in your body to get higher properly. Pay interest to how your frame feels, take time for self-care, and hold in thoughts that healing is simply as vital as staying lively to reap your health desires nicely and correctly.

The Role of Nutrition in Senior CrossFit

CrossFit is a incredible exercise application for human beings of every age, which incorporates seniors which includes you. We've talked about the significance of starting with a baseline assessment earlier than diving into CrossFit. Now, permit's delve deeper into a few component similarly important: your nutrients. What you eat plays a huge function in how properly you carry out, get higher, and live healthy. In this positive exploration, we are going to spread why vitamins holds paramount significance in senior CrossFit and the right guidelines you need to maintain in mind to optimize your workout workout routines.

The Foundation of Senior CrossFit Nutrition

Good nutrients serves because the foundational cornerstone for a sturdy and effective exercising software, and this holds actual for CrossFit, too. Choosing the right substances can increase your typical performance, lessen the chance of harm, aid in muscle recuperation, and contribute to everyday fitness. Let's dissect the important thing dietary components you need to carefully recall as a senior undertaking CrossFit.

1. Balancing Your Nutrients: Focus on a nicely-balanced food regimen that consists of the proper combo of carbohydrates, protein, and wholesome fats. Carbohydrates provide the energy critical, specially sooner or later of immoderate-depth CrossFit bodily sports. Protein helps muscle maintenance and regeneration, while healthy fat make contributions to regular health. Consider beginning your day with a mixture of complete-grain oats (carbs), Greek yogurt (protein), and a handful of almonds (excellent fats) to hold energy at a few level within the morning.

2. Staying Hydrated: Hydration is of most significance, mainly in the direction of strenuous activities like CrossFit. Monitoring fluid intake is essential to save you dehydration, which can cause cramps and dwindled feature. Ensure you live hydrated thru using sipping water at a few degree inside the day, and keep in thoughts incorporating a sports activities activities

drink with electrolytes at some point of your CrossFit lessons.

3. Timing Your Nutrients: Pay hobby to at the same time as you eat your meals. Post-workout, a aggregate of carbohydrates and protein aids in replenishing glycogen degrees and permits muscle restore. A placed up-exercising smoothie with protein powder and a banana is an exceptional desire to provide the essential protein and carbs for recuperation.

4. Eating Micronutrient-Rich Foods: Senior CrossFit participants ought to prioritize a diet plan rich in nutrients and minerals as the ones are crucial for everyday health and damage prevention. For example, calcium is critical for retaining bone fitness, which will become an increasing number of important with age. Foods together with leafy veggies, dairy merchandise, and fortified devices can contribute to meeting the ones dietary needs.

5. Managing Caloric Intake: Seniors want to take look at in their caloric intake to make

sure they have got enough strength for each CrossFit exercising workouts and each day sports sports. Seeking steerage from a licensed nutritionist can help have a take a look at man or woman calorie requirements, thinking about factors which encompass interest degree, goals, and everyday health.

6. Considering Supplements: In incredible times, seniors may also gain from nutritional nutritional nutritional supplements to cope with specific dietary deficiencies, in particular if there are nutritional policies or health issues. Consulting with healthcare professionals can manual seniors on the right use of diet or mineral supplements.

7. Adapting to Changing Needs: Aging can result in changes in nutritional desires, which incorporates a decline in urge for meals or alterations in digestion. Seniors ought to be aware of those changes and alter their food behavior because of this. Opting for nutrient-dense and resultseasily digestible foods,

which include lean meats, boiled greens, and moderate fruits, can be a wise desire.

eight. Special Dietary Considerations: Seniors may also have specific dietary dreams because of scientific situations or medication utilization. To address those character necessities, it's far critical to speak over with healthcare experts. For example, a senior with diabetes should cautiously control carbohydrate intake and show display screen blood sugar tiers in the course of CrossFit sporting events.

Nutrition serves as a linchpin inside the realm of senior CrossFit. Making knowledgeable and conscientious food alternatives offers the electricity, useful resource, and restoration essential for fulfillment on this demanding schooling application. Seniors need to area emphasis on maintaining a balanced food plan wealthy in critical nutrients, staying hydrated, considering nutrient timing, managing calorie consumption, adapting to converting dietary goals, and addressing unique concerns. By integrating those nutritional concepts into their way of life, seniors taking part in CrossFit can increase their normal overall performance, decorate their normal fitness, and acquire the manifold advantages of this dynamic exercising software program software.

Recovery Techniques for Senior Athletes

As seniors increasingly encompass CrossFit, recognizing the importance of effective healing techniques turns into paramount. These recuperation strategies extend beyond simply enhancing overall performance; they feature vital equipment in minimizing harm dangers and ensuring sustained engagement in CrossFit schooling over the lengthy haul. This complete guide targets to shed mild on numerous healing strategies mainly designed for senior CrossFit fans, providing centered insights to help you maintain not in reality physical fitness however furthermore the motivation to live active.

Active Recovery: On days while immoderate-intensity workout workouts aren't at the agenda, do not forget incorporating low-depth sporting activities into your ordinary. Activities collectively with gentle yoga, swimming, or leisurely walks can stimulate blood go together with the float, alleviate muscular soreness, and beautify common mobility without subjecting your body to undue stress.

Foam Rolling and Self-Myofascial Release (SMR): Embrace the exercise of froth rolling and self-myofascial release the use of gadget like foam rollers or lacrosse balls. This targeted method aids in relieving muscle tension, addressing knots or cause factors, and promoting superior flexibility. For example, incorporating a couple of minutes of froth rolling post a traumatic CrossFit consultation can contribute substantially to easing muscle tension, specially in regions like quadriceps and calf muscle corporations.

Nutrition and Hydration: The feature of vitamins inside the restoration procedure cannot be overstated. For superior muscle repair and glycogen replenishment, preserve a properly-balanced diet regime wealthy in protein and carbohydrates. Adequate hydration is similarly important, as dehydration can result in muscle cramps and dwindled ordinary overall overall performance. After a CrossFit consultation, recollect a positioned up-workout snack comprising lean protein property like hen or tofu and complex carbohydrates together with brown rice or quinoa.

Sleep and Rest: Prioritize an extremely good night's sleep, as it serves as a important element of the recovery manner. Aim for 7-nine hours of uninterrupted sleep every night time to permit your body to repair and renew tissues. Equally critical is incorporating enough relaxation among excessive training periods to prevent overtraining. Establishing a steady sleep routine and developing a relaxing bedtime ritual can make a contribution to more restful sleep.

Stretching and Mobility Work: Focusing on maintaining flexibility is vital for senior athletes to save you injuries and decorate ordinary mobility. Regular incorporation of stretching and mobility physical video video games into your regular can decorate kind of motion, alleviate muscle stiffness, and sell joint health. Implementing static stretches focused on key muscle groups, which encompass hips and shoulders normally engaged in CrossFit sports activities, can be beneficial.

Cold Water Immersion: Experiment with bloodless water immersion or assessment baths, alternating among heat and cold water. When accomplished cautiously and considering any underlying clinical conditions, those practices may additionally assist in lowering inflammation and muscular ache. For instance, a brief bloodless bathe or the utility of bloodless packs to precise muscle areas after an excessive CrossFit workout can useful resource in minimizing infection.

Professional Assistance: Seek the steering of healthcare experts, in conjunction with bodily therapists, chiropractors, or rubdown therapists. These professionals can provide tailored advice, strategies for addressing particular demanding situations, and make sure your regular fitness and protection. A consultation with a bodily therapist, as an example, also can assist alleviate recurrent joint pain or mobility boundaries.

Mind-Body Techniques: Incorporate strain-bargain strategies collectively with mindfulness and meditation into your healing recurring. These practices make a contribution not handiest to stress control however moreover to intellectual nicely-being and ordinary restoration. A brief meditation or mindfulness session included into your every day normal can function a valuable tool in handling strain and selling recovery.

Supportive Gear: Explore the benefits of carrying supportive gadget, which consist of compression garb or braces. These aids can expedite the recuperation approach with the beneficial aid of enhancing blood drift, minimizing muscle swelling, and imparting joint balance. Utilizing compression sleeves on legs or arms in a few unspecified time within the future of and after a CrossFit consultation, as an instance, can contribute to preventing muscle pain and swelling.

Listening to the Body: Perhaps the most critical approach is to actively pay attention in your body. Pay interest to any signals of ache or ache, and be willing to adjust your schooling due to this. Allow your self the strength to rest while desired and avoid pushing via immoderate fatigue or ache. If experiencing recurrent joint ache, undergo in thoughts editing or omitting unique movements and are attempting to find advice from a teach or healthcare practitioner.

Chapter 9: Cross Match

Assessing Your Fitness Level

In order to embark on a successful health adventure, it's far critical to evaluate your present day fitness degree. This will assist you region realistic dreams and create a custom designed workout plan that meets your wishes and abilities. Whether you're a pupil trying to beautify your ordinary health, an character looking for to shed kilos via Cross fit, or a person recuperating from an damage, this chapter will manual you via the technique of assessing your fitness stage.

Before diving into any fitness software, it's far critical to speak over with a healthcare expert, mainly when you have any underlying fitness conditions or modern-day accidents. Once you have got received the green mild, you can start through evaluating your cardiovascular staying electricity, energy, flexibility, and body composition.

Cardiovascular endurance is a key element of normal health. You can determine this thru appearing sports activities that improve your heart rate, which consist of walking or jumping rope. Keep music of methods prolonged you can preserve the ones sports activities and the manner speedy your heart fee recovers after exertion.

Strength evaluation can be finished thru bodily video games like push-ups, squats, and planks. Start with some repetitions and gradually increase the depth as you development. This will assist you find out which muscle agencies need more interest and set energy goals for this reason.

Flexibility is often unnoticed, however it performs a important characteristic in conventional health and damage prevention. Simple stretches like touching your toes or doing shoulder rotations can give you an idea of your modern-day flexibility level.

Body composition assessment consists of figuring out your percentage of body fat rather than muscle corporations. While there are expert strategies to be had, a clean technique is to use a body fats caliper or degree your waist circumference. This will help you track changes to your body composition as you progress for your fitness journey.

Remember, assessing your health diploma isn't always about comparing yourself to others. It is ready knowledge in which you are starting from and where you need to move. By comparing your cardiovascular persistence, power, flexibility, and body composition, you may set practical goals and create a tailor-made Crossfit software that suits your desires. Whether you are a novice, looking for weight reduction, or recuperating from an harm, taking the time to evaluate your health degree will lay the inspiration for a a hit and stable health journey.

Finding a Crossfit Box

One of the primary steps to embarking in your CrossFit journey is finding the proper CrossFit field for you. A CrossFit box is a specialized health club that gives CrossFit education and a supportive community of like-minded people. Whether you are a scholar, a health enthusiast, or a person looking to shed pounds or save you accidents, locating the ideal CrossFit difficulty will set you up for success.

When trying to find a CrossFit field, there are a few key factors to do not forget. Firstly, vicinity is critical. Look for a field that is with no trouble located near your house, place of business, or university. This will make it much less hard with a purpose to comprise CrossFit into your each day ordinary without any extra tour time.

Next, take a close to take a look at the centers and device available at every vicinity. CrossFit sporting activities frequently require a number of device, collectively with barbells, kettlebells, and pull-up bars. Ensure that the sphere you select has a properly-prepared facility with enough system to residence your desires.

Another essential problem to recall is the training group of workers. CrossFit sporting activities may be immoderate and require proper form and method to prevent accidents. Look for a area with professional and certified coaches who can guide you via the physical sports and provide personalised interest. This is mainly crucial in case you are a newbie or have any present accidents or rehabilitation wishes.

Furthermore, don't forget the elegance time table and environment of the field. Some boxes offer unique instructions for novices or weight reduction, at the equal time as others cater to a more competitive crowd. Determine which environment aligns together together with your goals and choices. Additionally, take a look at if the field offers bendy elegance instances that during form some time desk.

Lastly, recall to take charge beneath interest. CrossFit memberships can range in fee, so recall your rate range and the value you may be getting from the world. Some containers offer more centers collectively with vitamins steering or vicinity of understanding commands, which may be worth the greater charge for you.

Overall, finding the right CrossFit container is essential to beginning your health adventure at the right foot. Consider elements which encompass location, facilities, training personnel, class time desk, and price even as making your decision. Remember, a supportive community and informed coaches will play a massive feature to your fulfillment and amusement of CrossFit. So, take some time, go to awesome boxes, and discover the only that looks as if the proper healthful for you.

Crossfit Equipment and Apparel

When it entails Crossfit, having the proper device and clothing is crucial for a a achievement and amusing workout. Whether you are a beginner, someone trying to shed kilos, or an character centered on rehabilitation and harm prevention, the right system could make all the difference in your Crossfit journey.

For novices, it's miles essential to start with the basics. Comfortable and breathable apparel is a need to, as Crossfit workout sporting events can be excessive and sweat-inducing. Opt for materials that wick away moisture to maintain you cool and dry for the duration of your exercising. Additionally, making an investment in an excellent pair of bypass-education footwear is crucial. These shoes offer the essential assist and stability for the severa actions and carrying activities worried in Crossfit.

If weight loss is your reason, there are particular device and apparel options that may useful useful resource to your journey. Consider incorporating a weighted vest into your sporting activities. Wearing a weighted vest gives resistance and intensity for your physical sports, helping to burn greater electricity and construct energy. Additionally, compression garb can provide advantages together with progressed motion and muscle manual, enhancing your average performance and helping in weight reduction efforts.

For the ones focusing on rehabilitation and harm prevention, certain device and apparel selections can assist protect and guide the frame. Investing in an excellent pair of knee sleeves or braces can provide balance and compression to the knee joint, lowering the risk of harm. Similarly, wrist wraps can offer extra manual for the wrists throughout movements that put pressure in this area. Foam rollers and lacrosse balls also are vital tools for self-myofascial launch, supporting to alleviate muscle tightness and save you injuries.

Regardless of your specific dreams within the realm of Crossfit, it is crucial to prioritize protection and luxury whilst selecting machine and garb. Always select items that in shape well and are appropriate for the kind of workout you may be doing. Remember,

Crossfit is a flexible and dynamic fitness utility, and having the proper gear will no longer best beautify your normal performance but moreover preserve you advocated and devoted in your fitness adventure.

Safety Considerations in Crossfit

CrossFit has won big reputation in latest years, attracting a massive type of human beings, collectively with university students, health lovers, and the general public. However, like every form of exercise, CrossFit comes with its very own set of protection considerations that need to no longer be disregarded. Whether you're a amateur, attempting to find weight loss, or enhancing from an harm, knowledge those safety measures is crucial to making sure a steady and effective CrossFit adventure.

For novices, it's miles essential to begin slow and regularly boom the depth of your sports activities. CrossFit exercising workouts are diagnosed for his or her immoderate intensity and sundry moves, which may be hard for those new to the regime. Prioritize mastering proper form and approach earlier than trying heavier weights or advanced sporting sports activities. Working with an authorized CrossFit train or trainer can provide beneficial guidance and assist prevent accidents.

Weight loss is a common intention for lots human beings accomplishing CrossFit. While the intensity of the sporting activities can be beneficial for losing kilos, it is vital to method weight reduction in a healthful and sustainable way. Maintaining a balanced food regimen, staying hydrated, and permitting particular sufficient rest and healing are key factors in accomplishing your weight reduction desires accurately. Pushing yourself too difficult or neglecting proper nutrition can lead to fatigue, muscle pressure, or perhaps more important fitness issues.

CrossFit additionally may be a valuable device for rehabilitation and harm prevention. However, it's miles crucial to artwork with a certified teach or trainer who can tailor the sports to suit your precise desires. If you've got a pre-cutting-edge harm or medical situation, it's miles critical to speak about with a healthcare expert earlier than embarking on a CrossFit software. They can provide notion into any adjustments or precautions you want to take to save you in addition harm and useful useful resource in your restoration device.

Regardless of your health desires, protection need to usually be a pinnacle precedence in CrossFit. Warm-up because it have to be before every exercise to prepare your body for the desires in advance and funky down afterward to promote muscle recuperation. Listen on your body and avoid pushing yourself beyond your limits, as this can growth the hazard of harm. If you enjoy ache or pain in the course of a workout, it is essential to prevent and are seeking out appropriate scientific interest if vital.

Remember, Cross Fit is a journey that calls for patience, patience, and willpower to safety. By following those safety worries, you can revel in the advantages of Cross Fit even as minimizing the hazard of harm, making it a in reality transformative enjoy for your health adventure.

Chapter 10: Cross Fit Fundamentals

Cross fit Terminology

In the arena of Cross Fit, there may be a completely specific language those units it aside from exceptional fitness disciplines. As a beginner, it's far vital to make yourself familiar with those terms to completely interact in and understand this dynamic health adventure. Whether you are attempting to shed pounds, rehabilitate from an damage, or certainly start your health adventure, this subchapter will offer you with the critical Cross Fit terminology to get began.

1. WOD: Short for "Workout of the Day," the WOD is the each day exercise prescribed via Cross Fit going for walks shoes. Each WOD is designed to check your electricity, persistence, and common fitness.

2. AMRAP: Stands for "As Many Rounds As Possible." In an AMRAP workout, you have been given a tough and rapid quantity of time to complete as many rounds of a specific set of bodily sports as you can.

3. Box: Refers to a Cross Fit health club. Unlike traditional gyms, Cross Fit bins are commonly smaller, community-oriented areas wherein contributors shape near-knit relationships.

4. Rx: Short for "prescribed." Completing a exercising "Rx" technique appearing it precisely as it's written, with none modifications or scaling.

5. Scaling: Adjusting the intensity or difficulty of a exercise to fit your modern-day fitness diploma. Scaling is essential for beginners, permitting you to frequently construct energy and endurance without risking damage.

6. PR: Abbreviation for "Personal Record Achieving a PR technique beating your preceding first-class performance in a particular exercising or exercise.

7. Macon: An immoderate-depth exercise that focuses on metabolic conditioning. Met cons generally incorporate a combination of

cardiovascular carrying events and weightlifting moves.

8. Double-under: A bounce rope exercises wherein the rope passes underneath your ft twice in a unmarried jump. Mastering double-under can substantially beautify your coordination and cardiovascular persistence.

9. Kipping: An approach applied in gymnastics-primarily based moves, which includes pull-united states and toes-to-bar that consists of producing momentum thru managed swinging motions.

10. Tabata: A form of high-intensity c programming language education (HIIT) that includes 20 seconds of immoderate workout located thru way of 10 seconds of rest, repeated for a whole of 4 mines.

By expertise the ones important Cross Fit terms, you will be organized to navigate your health adventure with self guarantee and correctly speak with trainers and fellow Cross Fitters. Remember, whether or not or now not or now not your aim is weight reduction, harm prevention, or normal health improvement, Cross Fit offers a severa and inclusive network that welcomes people of all backgrounds and skills. Embrace the undertaking and experience the adventure in the direction of a more healthy, more potent, and extra empowered you.

Basic Cross fit Movements

In this subchapter, we are able to delve into the fundamental movements that shape the backbone of Cross Fit training. Whether you are a pupil, a health fanatic, or someone on the lookout for to shed a few pounds, these easy moves will set you at the path to fulfillment on your Cross Fit journey. Additionally, if you have become higher from an harm or searching for to prevent one, gaining knowledge of the ones actions can appreciably contribute in your rehabilitation and damage prevention efforts.

1. Squats: Squats are one of the maximum essential movements in Cross Fit. They

interact numerous muscle agencies, which includes the quadriceps, hamstrings, glutes, and center. Whether you carry out air squats or improvement to weighted squats, this exercise strengthens your lower frame, improves mobility, and complements everyday stability.

2. Push-ups: Push-u.S.A.Are a fantastic higher body exercising that targets the chest, shoulders, triceps, and middle. They assist assemble pinnacle body strength and balance. For beginners, changed push-America of americamay be accomplished till enough electricity is superior to carry out a complete push-up.

3. Pull-ups: Pull-u.S. Of America of americawork the muscle tissues on your pinnacle frame, together with the decrease lower returned, shoulders, and arms. They are excellent for constructing power and are fairly powerful in improving grip power. If you aren't able to perform a whole pull-up to

begin with, assisted pull-up variations may be employed to step by step collect electricity.

4. Deadlights: Deadlights inside the important aim the muscle tissues on your lower once more, glutes, and hamstrings. They are exquisite for building common electricity and growing a stable basis for distinct movements. Learning proper shape and approach is important to save you accidents.

5. Burpees: Burpees are a entire-body exercising that combines factors of aerobic, energy, and staying energy. They goal more than one muscle organizations, enhance cardiovascular health, and help burn power. They can be modified based totally mostly on health level, making them appropriate for beginners and people looking to shed pounds.

These easy Cross Fit actions lay the groundwork for added advanced wearing activities and exercising exercises. Remember, proper form and approach is key to maximizing the blessings of these moves whilst minimizing the danger of harm.

Gradually growing depth and incorporating these movements into your normal will make contributions to weight loss, rehabilitation, and damage prevention.

Whether you are a scholar, a fitness fanatic, or a person looking for to improve their popular nicely-being, studying those fundamental movements will set you at the right path to reaching your health dreams via Cross Fit.

Importance of Proper Form and Technique

Proper shape and approach are the foundation of any a achievement fitness adventure, in particular in phrases of Cross fit. Whether you're a student, a person looking to shed kilos, or seeking rehabilitation and damage prevention, expertise the importance of proper form and technique is important for achieving your fitness dreams efficaciously and successfully.

For novices, it is important to enlarge a sturdy foundation in right shape and technique.

Cross fit sporting activities comprise a substantial type of sensible actions, collectively with squats, deadlights, and overhead presses. By analyzing the best shape from the start, you will no longer nice reduce the danger of damage but additionally optimize the effectiveness of each exercising. Improper form can result in awful muscle recruitment and imbalances, hindering your improvement and potentially main to setbacks.

If your purpose is weight reduction, proper form and method are similarly vital. By appearing actions efficaciously, you engage the meant muscle groups more effectively, growing the calorie burn and common intensity of your exercises. Additionally, retaining right form all through your Cross fit schooling allows to enhance your posture and frame alignment, leading to better muscle stability and trendy body composition.

Proper form and method play a massive role in rehabilitation and damage prevention as well. Crossfit exercising exercises are designed to beautify electricity, flexibility, and mobility. By executing moves with right shape, you could goal unique areas of inclined component or damage competently and efficiently. Moreover, specializing in approach ensures that you are walking within your body's limits, reducing the risk of further damage and selling a faster recuperation.

To ensure right shape and method, its miles fantastically endorsed to are attempting to find steering from a qualified Cross fit teach or trainer. They can provide you with customized steering, corrections, and changes tailored on your goals and goals. Additionally, listening to your body is essential. Pay interest to any ache or ache within the route of physical sports activities, and do now not hesitate to alter or scale moves as needed.

In conclusion, whether or no longer or no longer you are a amateur, searching for weight reduction, or targeted on rehabilitation and harm prevention, knowledge and prioritizing proper shape and method is essential on your Cross fit journey. By getting to know the basics and executing moves correctly, you will not handiest decrease the hazard of harm however moreover optimize your outcomes, making sure a secure, powerful, and worthwhile health experience.

Scaling Options for Beginners

When embarking for your Cross fit journey, it's far important to undergo in mind that everyone starts off evolved at a specific fitness degree. Cross fit a hundred and one: A Beginner's Guide to Starting Your Fitness Journey is designed to help university students and the general public navigates their manner through the sector of Cross fit. In this subchapter, we're successful to speak scaling alternatives for novices that specialize in considered one of kind niches which includes Cross fit for novices, Cross fit for weight reduction, and Cross fit for rehabilitation and harm prevention.

Cross fit for Beginners:

Starting a few issues new may be intimidating, especially as regards to health. Cross fit is not any exception. However, the beauty of Cross fit lies in its scalability. Beginners have to attention on getting to know the crucial actions and gradually developing depth. Scaling alternatives together with lowering weights, editing movements, or lowering repetitions permit novices to construct strength and self guarantee on the same time as minimizing the threat of harm. The secret's to begin small, listen to your body, and development at your personal pace.

Cross fit for Weight Loss:

Cross fit can be a remarkable tool for weight loss, as it combines excessive-intensity exercising workouts with functional actions. To efficaciously shed pounds, novices must awareness on incorporating aerobic-based totally exercising routines that increase coronary heart price and burn strength.

Scaling alternatives for weight reduction may encompass c programming language schooling, enhancing moves to growth depth, and incorporating metabolic conditioning wearing sports. With consistency and strength of will, Cross fit will assist you to collect your weight reduction desires.

Cross fit for Rehabilitation and Injury Prevention:

One of the incredible benefits of Cross fit is its functionality to assist humans get over accidents and save you future ones. Scaling alternatives for rehabilitation and harm prevention involve working carefully with running shoes or coaches who can manual you via modified movements and sports. By focusing on proper shape, controlled movements, and steadily growing depth, Cross fit can useful resource in recuperation and enhance susceptible regions to prevent future injuries.

Remember, scaling isn't a sign of weak factor, but instead a clever approach to make sure protection and gold fashionable improvement. As a novice, it's vital to prioritize approach and step by step boom intensity as your body adapts. Cross fit 101: A Beginner's Guide to Starting Your Fitness Journey gives a whole evaluation of scaling options and techniques, assisting you navigate your manner through the sector of Cross fit.

Whether you're a scholar or a member of the general public, this subchapter desires to empower you to embark for your Cross fit adventure with self belief. By information scaling alternatives for novices, human beings can tailor their exercise exercises to their particular wishes, whether it is for weight reduction, rehabilitation, or absolutely beginning their health adventure.

Chapter 11: Cross fit Workouts for Beginners

Warm-up and Mobility Exercises

In the arena of Cross fit, heat-up and mobility physical video games play a vital position in preparing your frame for the acute workout exercises in advance. Whether you are a amateur or a person seeking to shed kilos, rehabilitate an harm, or save you in addition accidents, incorporating right warmth-up and mobility sports sports into your routine is vital.

Before diving into any severe physical interest, its miles crucial to get your frame warmed up. This allows growth blood goes with the flow, beautify your middle body temperature, and prepare your muscular tissues and joints for the approaching exercise. A warmness-up consultation generally lasts round 10-15 mins and consists of dynamic sports activities that concentrate on essential muscle organizations.

Some effective warmness-up bodily sports embody on foot or biking to get your heart price up, arm and leg swings to loosen up the joints, and body weight actions like squats, lunges, and push-americato set off the muscle mass. These wearing sports activities now not best growth flexibility but additionally beautify your style of movement, permitting you to perform the wearing sports with better shape and performance.

Mobility sports activities sports are in addition critical, specifically for novices and those getting better from an damage. These physical video games focus on improving joint mobility, flexibility, and balance. Incorporating mobility physical sports into your regular can considerably lessen the chance of harm and decorate your normal overall performance.

Common mobility physical sports embody foam rolling, which permits release tension inside the muscles and growth blood drift, in addition to sports like hip openers, shoulder circles, and spinal twists to aim particular regions of the body. These bodily sports now not most effective beautify your sort of motion however moreover decorate your frame's potential to get better and adapt to the desires of Cross fit exercise exercises.

For those searching for to shed pounds, warm-up and mobility carrying sports are essential in getting geared up your frame for immoderate-intensity exercising exercises. By growing your coronary heart price and activating your muscular tissues, those bodily sports activities assist you burn extra power within the course of your exercise durations, ultimately assisting in weight reduction.

Similarly, for humans rehabilitating a damage, warm-up and mobility physical sports are critical in selling healing, preventing in addition damage, and restoring complete range of movement. These carrying activities may be tailor-made to aim precise areas of the body, permitting you to grade by grade regain energy and versatility.

In give up, regardless of your health dreams, incorporating warmth-up and mobility carrying sports into your Cross fit recurring is critical. By nicely making organized your frame for the acute physical activities, you may beautify your regular performance, save you injuries, and optimize your ordinary fitness journey. Remember, searching after your body is a critical part of engaging in your health desires, and heat-up and mobility sports are the foundation of that care.

Sample Cross fit Workouts for Beginners

In this subchapter, we will discover a range of pattern Cross fit workout workouts specifically designed for novices. Whether you are a scholar in search of to beautify your regular fitness or a member of the overall public trying to find effective workout physical activities, those workout workouts will serve as a splendid start line on your Cross fit journey. Additionally, in case you are interested in Cross fit for weight reduction or rehabilitation and harm prevention, those physical activities can be tailor-made to fit your specific dreams and dreams.

Workout 1: Bodyweight Circuit

This exercising makes a specialty of constructing power and patience the use of your personal body weight. Perform each exercise for 30 seconds with a 15-2d rest in among. Complete three rounds.

Squats

Push-ups

Lunges

Plank

Burpees

Workout 2: Cardio Blast

For those looking for to burn energy and shed kilos, this cardio-targeted workout is ideal. Perform every exercise for 45 seconds with a 20-2nd rest in between. Complete four rounds.

Jumping jacks

High knees

Mountain climbers

Jump squats

Bicycle crunches

Workout three: Rehabilitation and Injury Prevention

If you've got grow to be better from an harm or seeking to prevent destiny injuries, this exercising will assist enhance flexibility, balance, and not unusual power. Perform each exercising for forty five seconds with a 20-2nd rest in between. Complete three rounds.

Glute bridges

Bird dogs

Side planks

Clamshells

Single-leg deadlights

Remember, it's far critical to warmth up earlier than any workout and take note of your frame at some point of. Start with lighter weights or adjustments if desired, grade by grade progressing as you become more cushty and confident.

By incorporating the ones sample Cross fit workout routines into your normal, you may progressively build strength, enhance cardiovascular health, and obtain your desired dreams. Whether you are a student, a member of the general public, or a person looking for weight reduction or rehabilitation, Cross fit gives a flexible and powerful fitness approach for all. Stay triggered, live ordinary, and revel in the adventure within the route of a more healthful and additional fit your needs!

Please take a look at that it also includes advocated to discuss with a healthcare expert or licensed Cross fit instructor earlier than beginning any new exercise software, in particular if you have pre-existing clinical situations or injuries.

Bodyweight Workout

One of the crucial factor factors of Cross fit training is the ability to apply your very own frame weight to perform a huge style of carrying activities. Whether you're a student in search of to stay wholesome on a price variety or a current-day person looking for an effective exercise ordinary, frame weight wearing activities are a fantastic manner to get commenced to your health adventure. In this subchapter, we will find out the blessings of bodyweight workout routines and offer a entire guide to help you include them into your Cross fit training.

Cross fit for Beginners:

For beginners, bodyweight exercising exercises are an great start line. These wearing activities will let you growth a strong foundation of energy, coordination, and mobility, which might be critical for progressing to greater advanced actions. By mastering body weight sporting sports activities which include squats, push-ups, and lunges, you can build a robust base to improvement closer to extra hard workout routines.

Cross fit for Weight Loss:

If weight reduction is your purpose, body weight workouts can be a activity-changer. These wearing sports engage more than one muscle groups concurrently, ensuing in a immoderate calorie burn and improved metabolic rate. Additionally, frame weight moves like burgees, mountain climbers, and leaping jacks growth your coronary heart price, promoting fats burning and cardiovascular fitness. By combining body weight exercising workouts with a balanced diet regime, you can benefit wonderful weight reduction and beautify your well-known health stage.

Cross fit for Rehabilitation and Injury Prevention:

Bodyweight wearing sports activities are also useful for human beings getting better from accidents or attempting to find to prevent them. Unlike weightlifting bodily sports, frame weight sports located less pressure on your joints even as although imparting a difficult exercise. Whether you are rehabilitating from a sports activities sports activities harm or actually need to strengthen your muscle organizations and beautify flexibility, body weight bodily video games like planks, bridges, and leg increases assist you to regain energy and balance.

Incorporating Bodyweight Workouts into Your Routine:

To incorporate frame weight workout workouts into your Cross fit recurring, begin by way of manner of identifying your health dreams. Whether you're a newbie, aiming for weight loss, or that specialize in rehabilitation, select out sports that align collectively along with your targets. Begin with vital moves and step by step progress to greater superior variations as your electricity and potential beautify. Remember to heat up well, hold tremendous form in the direction of each workout, and pay attention to your frame to keep away from damage.

In end, body weight exercise routines are a flexible and effective way to achieve numerous health dreams, making them appropriate for university youngsters and the overall public alike. Whether you are beginning your health adventure, aiming for weight reduction, or searching for rehabilitation and damage prevention, incorporating frame weight bodily video games into your Cross fit regular will yield sizable consequences. So clutch a mat, easy some region, and get prepared to assignment your frame and redesign your health degree with those effective and reachable sporting activities.

Dumbbell Workout

In the world of fitness, dumbbells are frequently underestimated, but they may be a powerful device in mission your health desires. Whether you are a scholar looking for to decorate normal electricity and regular overall performance, a member of the overall public searching for a ultra-modern exercise habitual, or a person inquisitive about CrossFit for weight reduction, rehabilitation, or harm prevention, incorporating dumbbells into your health habitual can yield exquisite results.

For novices in the realm of CrossFit, dumbbells provide a flexible and reachable choice. They are clean to use, require minimal vicinity, and offer a considerable variety of bodily sports that target top notch muscle businesses. With proper steerage and form, dumbbell wearing sports allow you to gather a stable foundation of electricity and endurance, preparing you for additonal immoderate CrossFit moves that lie in advance.

If your fitness adventure includes weight reduction, dumbbell bodily games may be rather effective. By appearing compound bodily games that interact more than one muscle groups concurrently, you can burn greater energy and raise your metabolism. With ordinary dumbbell schooling, you'll not only shed undesirable kilos but additionally sculpt and tone your frame, developing a lean and defined body.

For those rehabilitating from an damage or looking for damage prevention, dumbbell workout sports are an first-rate preference. They assist you to isolate and enhance precise muscle agencies, assisting within the healing method and decreasing the risk of similarly damage. Additionally, dumbbells sell stability and stability, important factors for damage prevention, making sure which you keep proper shape and alignment for the duration of exercising workouts.

To maximize the advantages of a dumbbell workout, it is critical to layout a nicely-rounded routine. This might in all likelihood include bodily video video games collectively with dumbbell squats, lunges, shoulder presses, bicep curls, and tricep extensions, amongst others. It is crucial to start with lighter weights and step by step growth the weight as your electricity improves.

Remember, protection is paramount at the equal time as incorporating dumbbells into your fitness ordinary. Always warmth up because it must be earlier than exercising, maintain right shape for the duration of each movement, and pay attention in your body. If you're unsure approximately right approach or want guidance, searching for recommendation from a certified CrossFit educate or private instructor.

In end, dumbbell workout exercises are a treasured addition to any fitness journey, whether or now not or not you are a scholar, a member of the general public, or in search of precise dreams collectively with weight reduction, rehabilitation, or damage prevention. By incorporating dumbbells into your routine, you could decorate your normal energy, burn electricity, sculpt your frame, and sell balance and balance. So grasp those dumbbells, get moving, and embark on your CrossFit adventure these days!

Kettlebell Workout

One of the simplest device in a CrossFit workout is the kettlebell. This versatile piece of system has been used for hundreds of years and is a staple in lots of health workouts. In this subchapter, we are capable of explore the blessings of incorporating kettlebell physical activities into your CrossFit education, whether you are a amateur looking for to begin your health adventure, aiming for weight loss, or looking for rehabilitation and damage prevention.

For beginners, kettlebell bodily sports provide an brilliant creation to CrossFit. They provide a entire-body exercising that goals multiple muscle companies concurrently. The dynamic movements completed with kettlebells help to enhance power, staying strength, and coordination. With proper method and steering from a certified CrossFit educate, beginners can fast studies the basics and development to greater complicated moves.

If weight reduction is your goal, the kettlebell is an first-rate device to comprise into your normal. Kettlebell physical games are recounted for his or her immoderate-intensity nature, which lets in to burn a big amount of energy in a brief period. The swinging and lifting motions have interaction the entire frame, boosting your metabolism and promoting fat loss. Additionally, kettlebell carrying sports assemble lean muscle mass, which further increases your metabolic charge and permits you burn more electricity in some unspecified time in the future of the day.

For those improving from an harm or attempting to find to save you destiny injuries, kettlebell carrying activities can be a activity-changer. The managed actions achieved with kettlebells assist to enhance stabilizing muscle businesses, decorate stability, and beautify flexibility. The kettlebell's particular shape and grip furthermore make contributions to constructing grip energy, it certainly is crucial for supporting joints and preventing common accidents.

In this subchapter, we are capable of provide a entire guide to kettlebell sporting sports suitable for beginners, those aiming for weight loss, and individuals searching out rehabilitation and damage prevention. We will communicate right shape and technique, endorsed weights, and improvement techniques. Additionally, we will cope with common mistakes and offer recommendations for keeping off accidents.

Whether you're a pupil or a member of the general public, the kettle bell exercising subchapter in "CrossFit one zero one: A Beginner's Guide to Starting Your Fitness Journey" will characteristic a useful aid for incorporating this flexible tool into your fitness habitual. No rely your fitness goals, kettlebell exercising workouts can provide the venture and results you desire, all even as improving your normal energy, staying power, and mobility.

Tracking and Progressing in Crossfit

Tracking and progressing in Crossfit is critical for novices, individuals on the lookout for to lose weight, and those in search of rehabilitation and harm prevention. By tracking your wellknown basic overall performance and making constant improvement, you may gain your health goals and enhance your not unusual properly-being.

For beginners, monitoring your exercising workouts permits you to look how a long manner you have come and offers motivation to preserve going. Start with the useful resource of the usage of recording your initial fitness diploma, which embody your weight, body measurements, and any electricity or staying power assessments. This baseline will function a reference factor for future improvement. As you preserve your Crossfit adventure, song your exercise workouts, noting the physical games, weights used, and the shape of repetitions or devices finished. This statistics will help you spot enhancements over time and find out regions that want more hobbies.

In addition to monitoring your exercising routines, it's far crucial to consciousness on progressing in Crossfit. This can be accomplished with the resource of the use of steadily developing the intensity, duration, or resistance of your sports activities activities. For weight loss, progressing in Crossfit is essential to constantly difficult your frame and burning electricity. By incorporating excessive-intensity interval schooling (HIIT) and compound movements, you could maximize your calorie burn and shed more kilos.

Chapter 12: Cross Fit for Weight Loss

How Cross fit Can Help with Weight Loss

One of the primary reasons why humans gravitate toward Cross fit is its effectiveness in promoting weight loss. In this subchapter, we're capable of delve into the strategies Cross fit can assist humans shed the ones more pounds and benefit their weight loss goals.

First and vital, Cross fit exercising workouts are designed to be immoderate-depth and continuously various, because of this that they're in particular tailor-made to burn strength and fat. Unlike traditional gym exercises that concentrate on isolated muscle agencies, Cross fit exercise physical games have interaction the entire frame, resulting in a more calorie burn in some unspecified time in the future of and after each session. This elevated metabolic price is essential for weight reduction because it allows your frame to preserve burning calories even prolonged after you have left the gym.

Moreover, Cross fit sporting events comprise a combination of cardiovascular wearing occasions, weightlifting, and body weight movements. This severa variety of sporting occasions permits to construct lean muscular tissues while simultaneously growing your cardiovascular staying strength. The greater lean muscle you have were given, the higher your metabolism becomes, which translates to greater electricity burned at a few stage in the day.

In addition to the physical advantages, Cross fit moreover emphasizes proper vitamins as an essential a part of the weight reduction adventure. The e-book "Cross fit 101: A Beginner's Guide to Starting Your Fitness Journey" offers treasured insights into the importance of vitamins and gives steering at the way to gas your body for most beneficial weight reduction. By adopting a balanced and nutritious weight loss plan, you could enhance the effectiveness of your Cross fit sports activities and gather your weight reduction desires extra hastily.

Furthermore, Cross fit isn't quite an lousy lot losing weight; it is also approximately reworking your preferred life-style. The supportive and motivating network that surrounds Cross fit allows people stay committed to their fitness journey. Through shared research and encouragement, you'll find out the electricity to push past your limits and gain effects you by no means idea possible.

Whether you're a newbie seeking to start your health adventure, a person searching for weight reduction answers, or maybe an man or woman in need of rehabilitation or damage prevention, Cross fit can be tailor-made to suit your specific dreams. By taking element in Cross fit workout routines, you will no longer only shed undesirable pounds however also enjoy superior energy, staying electricity, and everyday well-being.

In conclusion, Cross fit is a particularly effective and green way to benefit weight loss. Its aggregate of excessive-depth exercise workout routines, numerous carrying activities, and attention on proper nutrients make it an exquisite preference for human beings looking for to shed those more pounds and rework their lives. So, why wait? Embrace the project and be a part of the Cross fit network nowadays!

Nutrition Tips for Cross fit and Weight Loss

Proper nutrients play a essential function in attaining most effective common performance and weight loss dreams in Cross fit. Whether you are a novice, looking for to shed a few kilos, or getting higher from an harm, following the ones vitamins guidelines will help you maximize your results and lead a more fit way of life.

1. Prioritize Whole Foods: Focus on ingesting whole, unprocessed components that provide essential vitamins. Incorporate lean proteins like hen, fish, and tofu, together with a number of forestall end result, veggies, complete grains, and wholesome fats. Avoid

sugary snacks, processed ingredients, and immoderate caffeine.

2. Eat Balanced Meals: Ensure that your meals include a stability of macronutrients carbohydrates, proteins, and fats. Carbohydrates provide power, proteins useful resource muscle repair and boom, and fat help not unusual fitness. Aim to embody all 3 in every meal to preserve solid power ranges and beautify healing.

3. Hydration is Key: Stay hydrated in advance than, sooner or later of, and after your workout exercises. Water is essential for maximum appropriate performance and aids in digestion, metabolism, and nutrient absorption. Carry a water bottle with you and sip regularly in a few unspecified time within the destiny of the day.

4. Pre and Post-Workout Nutrition: Fuel your frame earlier than and after each exercise to optimize common performance and healing. Prior to a exercise, consume effortlessly digestible carbohydrates like fruit or a small

serving of entire grains. After a exercising, fill up your glycogen shops through ingesting a combination of carbohydrates and protein internal 30 minutes.

5. Portion Control: Pay interest to element sizes to keep away from overeating. Use smaller plates and bowls to trick your thoughts into wondering you're eating a bigger element. Listen in your frame's hunger and fullness cues and devour till you are glad, no longer overly stuffed.

6. Meal Planning and Preparation: Plan your meals earlier to make sure you have got were given nutritious alternatives without issue available. Prepare food and snacks in bulk, and element them out to avoid impulsive and terrible food alternatives. This will maintain time and save you from conducting for quick, processed alternatives.

7. Seek Professional Guidance: Consult a registered dietitian or nutritionist to tailor your nutrients plan especially in your dreams and goals. They can provide custom designed

tips, help you conquer any nutritional stressful conditions, and show your development.

Remember, vitamins is surely as essential because the bodily aspect of Cross fit. By adopting these nutrients guidelines, you'll gas your frame for achievement, aid weight loss efforts, and decorate your regular properly-being.

Combining Cross fit with Other Forms of Exercise

When it includes accomplishing your health desires, incorporating an entire lot of physical sports into your habitual is crucial. Cross Fit, a excessive-depth health software program, can be a awesome basis for reinforcing your well-known health level. However, to maximize your results and save you burnout, it is crucial to combine Cross Fit with special kinds of exercising. Whether you are a amateur, looking to lose weight, or seeking out rehabilitation and damage prevention, integrating one-of-a-kind modalities can offer particular blessings tailored on your precise desires.

For Cross Fit novices, it is vital to understand that this system itself already consists of various sports. From weightlifting and cardio to gymnastics and realistic moves, Cross Fit offers a complete workout ordinary. However, supplementing your Cross Fit regular with other bodily games collectively with yoga or Pilates can help enhance flexibility, stability, and center energy. Additionally, inclusive of low-effect carrying activities like swimming or biking on relaxation days can aid in recuperation and prevent overtraining.

Chapter 13: Cross Fit for Rehabilitation and Injury Prevention

Cross fit for Injury Rehabilitation

In the sector of health, Cross Fit has received large popularity for its excessive-intensity workout routines and ability to push human beings to their limits. While it's far typically associated with weight loss and electricity constructing, CrossFit moreover boasts severa advantages for harm rehabilitation and prevention. In this subchapter, we're able to find out how CrossFit can be an powerful tool in convalescing from injuries and retaining a wholesome, energetic lifestyle.

When it involves damage rehabilitation, CrossFit gives a completely precise approach that focuses on beneficial movements and not unusual health. Unlike conventional rehabilitation techniques that isolate specific muscle agencies, CrossFit emphasizes full-body bodily sports that have interaction multiple muscle groups concurrently. This holistic method now not exceptional speeds up recovery however additionally lets in prevent destiny accidents thru strengthening the entire frame.

One of the key requirements of CrossFit is scalability, which means carrying activities may be tailor-made to character wishes and abilties. This makes it a fantastic preference for human beings recuperating from accidents, as sporting events may be modified or substituted to house boundaries. CrossFit coaches are nicely-knowledgeable in damage prevention and rehabilitation techniques, making sure that individuals carry out movements efficiently and efficiently.

Furthermore, the inclusive and supportive community element of CrossFit performs a crucial function in harm rehabilitation. The camaraderie and encouragement from fellow athletes may be substantially motivating in a few unspecified time within the destiny of the restoration technique. The shared studies and expertise within the CrossFit network also can provide valuable insights and recommendation for harm prevention and rehabilitation.

CrossFit's emphasis on practical actions is especially useful for those searching out rehabilitation. By incorporating movements that mimic regular sports, together with squatting, lifting, and pushing, human beings regain power and mobility that right away translates into their everyday lives. Additionally, the various and continuously converting workouts maintain individuals engaged and recommended, reducing the probabilities of boredom and making sure consistent improvement.

However, it is critical to be conscious that CrossFit for harm rehabilitation should be approached with warning and beneath the guidance of experts. Consulting with a healthcare corporation or physical therapist earlier than starting any CrossFit software program is especially recommended, as they may be able to provide precise pointers and changes primarily based totally on character desires.

In end, CrossFit isn't clearly confined to weight loss or power building; it could furthermore be a effective tool for harm rehabilitation and prevention. With its interest on useful moves, scalability, and supportive network, CrossFit can aid in a quick healing and help human beings regain their physical fitness and not unusual nicely-being. Whether you're a amateur or skilled, CrossFit gives a comprehensive method to fitness that caters to a huge sort of people, at the side of the ones looking for to rehabilitate from accidents.

Preventing Common Injuries in Crossfit

Crossfit has received mammoth recognition in current years, attracting college students and the overall public with its extreme and dynamic exercise workouts. However, like all health regime, it isn't always with out its risks. In order to make certain a secure and injury-unfastened Crossfit enjoy, it is essential to be aware of the not unusual injuries that could occur and take preventive measures to avoid them.

One of the maximum important elements of harm prevention in Crossfit is proper technique and form. Beginners regularly get stuck up within the excitement and depth of the workouts, neglecting proper shape and setting themselves at chance. It is crucial to start with a strong foundation, focusing on mastering the basic movements and gradually growing the depth.

Another key thing of harm prevention is listening to your frame. Pushing yourself to the boundaries is a fundamental precept of Crossfit, however it's miles equally vital to know your limits and keep away from overtraining. Rest and recuperation days are simply as crucial because the exercising days, as they permit your frame to heal and give a boost to. Ignoring fatigue and pushing thru pain can result in critical injuries that could set you back for weeks or even months.

Additionally, incorporating mobility and flexibility physical games into your regular routine can greatly reduce the threat of injuries. Crossfit includes a huge variety of movements and calls for flexibility and mobility in various joints and muscular tissues. Spending time on stretching and mobility sports earlier than and after workout routines can assist enhance your range of movement and prevent muscle traces and joint injuries.

For people trying to lose weight thru Crossfit, it is important to technique weight loss steadily and with caution. Rapid weight loss can placed immoderate pressure on your joints and growth the threat of injuries. Working with an authorized Crossfit instructs or private teacher who can guide you thru a safe and effective weight reduction adventure is enormously encouraged.

Lastly, for those who are the usage of Crossfit for rehabilitation and harm prevention, it's miles essential to talk openly with your coach or instructor about any pre-current injuries or barriers. They can regulate exercises and offer opportunity sports that will help you get better and prevent further accidents.

In end, Crossfit may be a notably powerful and rewarding fitness journey, but it's miles important to prioritize damage prevention. By that specialize in proper method, taking note of your frame, incorporating mobility physical games, and searching for steering when wanted, you may experience the benefits of Crossfit whilst minimizing the chance of common injuries. Remember, your health and safety has to always be the top precedence in any fitness undertaking.

Working with Physical Therapists and Coaches

When embarking on your fitness adventure, it's far vital to apprehend the importance of running with professionals who can manual and help you alongside the way. Physical therapists and coaches play a crucial role in assisting people obtain their health dreams, whether or not it's weight loss, rehabilitation, or damage prevention. In this subchapter, we are able to delve into the advantages of participating with these specialists, in particular within the context of Crossfit.

Crossfit for novices:

For folks who are new to Crossfit, the steering and knowledge of a physical therapist or teach could make all of the difference. They will investigate your modern fitness degree, become aware of any limitations or weaknesses, and layout a customized education program that suits your wishes. These specialists will ensure which you research proper form and approach for each exercise, lowering the threat of damage and maximizing your results. They will even offer ongoing guide and motivation, helping you stay on the right track and gain your dreams.

Chapter 14: Cross Fit Training Programs

Beginner's Cross fit Training Program

Cross fit one hundred and one: A Beginner's Guide to Starting Your Fitness Journey

Welcome to the world of Cross fit! Whether you are a pupil seeking to improve your normal health or a member of the overall public searching for a new and exciting workout routine, this beginner's Crossfit schooling program is designed to help you kickstart your health adventure. In this subchapter, we will cover the fundamentals of Crossfit for novices, as well as its ability benefits for weight loss, rehabilitation, and injury prevention.

Crossfit for Beginners:

Starting a brand new health program can be intimidating; however Crossfit presents supportive and inclusive surroundings for all health degrees. This schooling program will introduce you to crucial Crossfit actions, consisting of squats, deadlifts, push-ups, and pull-ups, even as progressively growing intensity and complexity over the years. It is vital to attention on right shape and method to save you accidents and build a stable basis for future exercises.

Crossfit for Weight Loss:

If weight loss is your number one purpose, Crossfit may be a recreation-changer. Combining excessive-intensity purposeful movements with cardiovascular sporting events, Crossfit facilitates you burn calories, boost your metabolism, and build lean muscular tissues. This program will incorporate a combination of strength education, cardio sports, and c language education to maximise fats loss and enhance usual body composition.

Crossfit for Rehabilitation and Injury Prevention:

One of the particular aspects of Crossfit is its scalability, which permits people with numerous health ranges and accidents to participate. This schooling software consists of changed physical games and opportunity moves that could resource in rehabilitation and harm prevention. Crossfit specializes in useful movements that improve joint balance, mobility, and normal electricity, helping you recover from accidents and save you destiny ones.

Remember, consistency is key in relation to any health program. This training application need to be approached with dedication and staying power. Progress can also range from person to person, but with consistent attempt, you will see improvements on your strength, endurance, and average health degree.

Before beginning any new exercising software, it is usually recommended to consult with a healthcare professional, especially when you have any pre-existing clinical situations or accidents. They can provide personalized steerage and make certain that you are schooling safely and correctly.

Get geared up to embark on an interesting fitness adventure with Crossfit! Whether you're a beginner trying to analyze the basics, aiming for weight loss, or searching for rehabilitation and harm prevention, this training program will help you achieve your fitness desires. Remember, Crossfit is greater than only a exercise, it is a network that supports and motivates you each step of the way.

Intermediate Crossfit Training Program

In this subchapter, we are able to delve into the sector of intermediate Crossfit training packages. Whether you are a student trying to take your health to the following stage or a member of the overall public keen to beautify your Crossfit adventure, this section will offer you with the steering and understanding you need to progress in your schooling.

Crossfit for Beginners:

For those who have mastered the fundamentals of Crossfit and are prepared to push their limits, intermediate schooling software is the ideal next step. This application specializes in building strength, staying power, and skill, at the same time as also incorporating more superior sporting events and techniques. By steadily increasing the intensity and complexity of your workouts, you'll preserve to assignment your frame and spot considerable upgrades in your universal fitness.

Crossfit for Weight Loss:

If weight loss is your primary goal, an intermediate Crossfit training program can be enormously powerful. By combining excessive-depth c program languageperiod schooling (HIIT) with functional movements, you may burn energy, construct lean muscle, and improve your metabolism. This application will also encompass sporting activities that concentrate on specific muscle businesses, supporting you tone and tighten your body even as dropping undesirable pounds.

Crossfit for Rehabilitation and Injury Prevention:

For people getting better from accidents or looking to save you them, an intermediate Crossfit software can offer a secure and powerful way to rebuild strength and versatility. This application wills consciousness on right shape and technique, step by step growing the weight and depth to ensure a slow and controlled progression. Additionally, incorporating mobility physical games and stretches will help prevent future injuries and enhance common joint fitness.

Throughout this subchapter, we will provide you with a number of intermediate Crossfit schooling exercises, designed to undertaking and inspire you. These packages will consist of a combination of electricity schooling, aerobic workouts, and talent development classes, ensuring a nicely-rounded and balanced technique on your health adventure.

Remember; always concentrate for your body and development at your personal tempo. Crossfit is set pushing your self, however it's equally important to prioritize safety and recuperation. With a dedicated mindset and commitment to your goals, an intermediate Crossfit schooling application will propel you towards new ranges of strength, endurance, and overall health.

Advanced Crossfit Training Program

For those who've already mastered the fundamentals of Crossfit and are equipped to take their health adventure to the subsequent stage, advanced schooling software can offer the undertaking and outcomes you searching for. This subchapter wills manual you thru a complicated Crossfit training program this is designed to push your limits and assist you acquire your fitness goals. Whether you're a scholar trying to improve your athletic performance or a member of the overall public in search of a brand new degree of physical fitness, this program has something to offer.

Crossfit for beginners laid the inspiration to your fitness adventure, and now it's time to build upon that foundation. This advanced schooling application introduces more complex movements and higher depth exercises to help you hold progressing. It is essential to observe that this program isn't always appropriate for beginners or people with certain fitness conditions. It is continually advocated to talk over with a healthcare expert earlier than starting any superior health software.

Chapter 15: Cross Fit Faqs and Troubleshooting

Addressing Common Concerns approximately Crossfit

CrossFit has gained big popularity through the years, attracting people from all walks of lifestyles who are trying to rework their fitness trips. However, it isn't always uncommon for ability novices to have issues or doubts approximately beginning CrossFit. In this subchapter, we can cope with some of the not unusual worries raised by using students and the general public, particularly specializing in CrossFit for beginners, CrossFit for weight loss, and CrossFit for rehabilitation and injury prevention.

One of the maximum common issues for beginners is the concern of no longer being in shape sufficient to begin CrossFit. It is critical to bear in mind that CrossFit is scalable, which means it could be adapted to any health level. Whether you are a pro athlete or just starting your fitness adventure, CrossFit can be changed to fit your desires and talents. Trained coaches are there to guide you through the system, ensuring that you progress at a tempo this is secured and effective.

Another issue frequently raised by means of people is the false impression that CrossFit is handiest for the ones seeking to construct bulky muscle groups. While electricity training is a giant element of CrossFit, it isn't always the only awareness. CrossFit workout routines are designed to improve average fitness, which includes factors which include cardiovascular patience, flexibility, and agility. These exercises are various and continuously numerous, ensuring that you never lose interest and that your body constantly adapts to new demanding situations.

For the ones interested in weight reduction, CrossFit may be an exceptional choice. The excessive-intensity nature of CrossFit exercises enables burn calories and builds lean muscle groups, which in turn will increase your metabolism even outside of the gymnasium. Additionally, the supportive community factor of CrossFit can provide the motivation and duty needed to gain your weight reduction goals.

Concerns about harm prevention and rehabilitation are legitimate, specifically for individuals who've had preceding accidents. It is essential to pick a good CrossFit gym with experienced coaches who prioritize protection. Coaches will make sure that you examine right form and method, reducing the risk of harm. Additionally, CrossFit may be an powerful device for rehabilitation under the guidance of a healthcare professional, because it emphasizes functional moves that may help enhance usual strength and mobility.

Dealing with Plateaus and Progress Stalls

In any fitness journey, it's miles not unusual to stumble upon plateaus and development stalls. These moments can be irritating and demotivating, however they're a herbal a part of the way. Understanding why plateaus arise and the way to triumph over them is vital for anyone embarking on a CrossFit journey. Whether you're a amateur, aiming for weight loss, or focused on rehabilitation and damage prevention, understanding the way to navigate those annoying situations will help you stay heading within the proper direction and attain your fitness desires.

Plateaus regularly get up while our bodies adapt to the workout every day we had been following. Initially, we also can experience fast upgrades in electricity, staying energy, or weight loss. However, as our our our bodies grow to be acquainted with the needs we location on them, progress can slow down or maybe come to a halt. This is while we want to rethink our education techniques and make essential modifications.

For novices in Cross Fit, plateaus can rise up while the body is not nicely organized for the depth of the exercise physical games. It is crucial to begin slowly and gradually growth the depth and length of your exercise workout routines. Additionally, specializing in right form and approach will assist prevent accidents and enhance wellknown accepted universal performance.

If weight loss is your purpose, you may enjoy plateaus at the same time as your body adapts to the caloric deficit or the exercising everyday you are following. To break via this plateau, keep in mind converting your workout ordinary, developing the depth, or incorporating new carrying sports. Additionally, reassessing your vitamins and ensuring you are ingesting a balanced diet regime can also help kickstart weight reduction yet again.

For human beings the use of CrossFit for rehabilitation and damage prevention, plateaus can be mainly irritating. It is crucial to art work carefully with a certified train or physical therapist that can layout a application tailor-made to your unique dreams. By focusing on targeted sports activities sports that deliver a boost to the injured region while additionally addressing desired fitness, you may gradually triumph over plateaus and maintain progressing closer to healing.

Regardless of the location of hobby you fall into, there are some present day strategies for overcoming plateaus and development stalls in CrossFit. Firstly, attempt numerous your physical games with the aid of way of the use of incorporating new physical games, changing the order of sports activities, or improving the depth. This will project your frame in new methods, preventing it from adapting and stagnating. Secondly, don't forget deloading or taking brief breaks from extreme workouts to permit your body to get better truely. Finally, preserve track of your progress, set realistic dreams, and feature an incredible time small victories along the way. This will help you live prompted and focused to your journey.

Remember, plateaus and progress stalls aren't signs and symptoms of failure however as an alternative possibilities for growth. By expertise the motives in the once more of those setbacks and enforcing the proper strategies, you could conquer them and preserve transferring forward to your Cross Fit adventure Stay dedicated, be affected individual, and enjoy the method of turning into stronger, more healthful, and extra wholesome.

Overcoming Mental Barriers in Crossfit

In the thrilling worldwide of Crossfit, wherein physical annoying situations push you on your limits, it's miles crucial to apprehend that the obstacles we often face aren't completely physical Our intellectual us of a plays a massive role in our capacity to prevail and accumulate our desires. In this subchapter, we're capable of discover the numerous intellectual limitations that novices, weight reduction lovers, and people trying to find rehabilitation and harm prevention can also stumble upon in their Crossfit adventure, and the manner to conquer them.

For novices, getting into a Crossfit gym can be intimidating. The fear of the unknown, the pressure to carry out, and the assessment to others may be overwhelming. The key to overcoming those mental limitations is to interest on your very non-public improvement and journey. Crossfit isn't always approximately competing with others; it's miles about pushing yourself to grow to be the tremendous model of yourself. Set practical goals, have a great time small victories, and surround yourself with a supportive community. Remember, each person starts someplace, and every expert changed into as soon as a newbie.

Chapter 16: Cross Fit Success Stories

Inspiring Crossfit Transformation Stories

In the arena of health, Crossfit has obtained huge recognition for its precise approach to training that mixes excessive-intensity sporting activities, useful movements, and a supportive community. This subchapter affords inspiring Crossfit transformation recollections that showcase the remarkable trips of people who have benefited from this fitness regimen. Whether you're a scholar looking for to enhance your usual fitness, a beginner in search of steering on starting your Crossfit journey, a person aiming for weight loss, or maybe someone rehabilitating from an damage, the ones stories are exceptional to encourage and inspire you.

First, permit's find out the transformation recollections of novices who have embraced Crossfit These people, like a number of us, have been to start with anxious approximately moving into a Crossfit container. However, via perseverance and the resource of their coaches and fellow athletes, they have got now not best finished their health dreams however moreover decided a newfound ardour for this sport. Their tales highlight the importance of beginning sluggish, being attentive to your frame, and trusting the approach.

For those searching for weight loss, Crossfit offers a whole application that mixes aerobic, power schooling, and nutrients. The recollections of people who've efficiently shed pounds through Crossfit will inspire you to push beyond your limits, make extra wholesome alternatives, and embody a greater lively way of life. These memories additionally emphasize the importance of motive putting, consistency, and the electricity of a supportive network in engaging in weight loss dreams.

Crossfit isn't simplest for novices or weight reduction lovers but moreover serves as an powerful device for rehabilitation and harm prevention. The recollections of individuals who've conquer accidents and regained their electricity through Crossfit display the transformative power of this health routine. From enhancing physical games to operating cautiously with coaches and physical therapists, those people have not most effective recovered however moreover grow to be more potent than ever in advance than.

In end, the inspiring Crossfit transformation recollections offered on this subchapter function a testomony to the giant capability of Crossfit for university students and the general public. Whether you are a amateur, looking for weight reduction, or improving from an damage, the ones reminiscences will encourage you to embark in your very private fitness adventure. Remember, Crossfit isn't quite plenty bodily transformation however additionally approximately constructing mental resilience and locating a supportive network if you want to push you to reap your goals. So, lace up your footwear, step proper into a Crossfit field, and put together to be amazed via manner of using the great adjustments that sit up for you.

Interviews with Crossfit Athletes

In this subchapter, we delve into the minds of professional CrossFit athletes who've excelled of their health adventure. Their insights and recollections will inspire and encourage each university college students and the general public who are inquisitive about CrossFit for beginners, weight reduction, rehabilitation, and harm prevention.

Interview 1: CrossFit for Beginners

We speak with Sarah, a CrossFit athlete who commenced her fitness adventure as a whole newbie. She stocks her traumatic conditions, triumphs, and advice for those just starting out. Sarah emphasizes the importance of taking it slow, specializing in right form, and frequently developing intensity. She furthermore discusses the supportive network she located within the CrossFit discipline and the manner it helped her live induced and accountable.

Interview 2: CrossFit for Weight Loss

In this interview, we talk to Mark, who efficiently misplaced a vast quantity of weight via CrossFit. He shares his transformation story and the way CrossFit no longer high-quality helped him shed kilos however additionally advanced his usual health and well-being. Mark gives pointers for incorporating CrossFit right proper into a weight loss journey, which includes the importance of nutrients, consistency, and placing practical goals.

Interview three: CrossFit for Rehabilitation and Injury Prevention

We communicate with Lisa, a CrossFit athlete who used CrossFit as a part of her rehabilitation way after a sports activities activities-associated damage. Lisa discusses how she worked closely at the side of her CrossFit educate and physical therapist to create a custom designed software that focused on strengthening her injured areas whilst preventing further injuries. She emphasizes the significance of listening to your frame, communicating collectively collectively with your teach, and steadily progressing to keep away from setbacks.

Throughout those interviews, we discover common subject matters that are applicable to all niches. These subjects embody the importance of proper shape, the strength of a supportive network, the need for regular attempt, and the information that development takes time. These interviews characteristic a reminder that CrossFit can be tailored to numerous health desires and levels, making it available to college students and the general public alike

www.ingramcontent.com/pod-product-compliance
Lightning Source LLC
Chambersburg PA
CBHW051726020426
42333CB00014B/1167